Keto Diet for Women Over 70

A Comprehensive Guide For Women To Discover Why Embracing the Ketogenic Lifestyle Is Never Too Late | Includes Quick and Tasty Recipes, a Meal Plan, an Exercise Plan & a Journal Diary

By

Melinda Francis

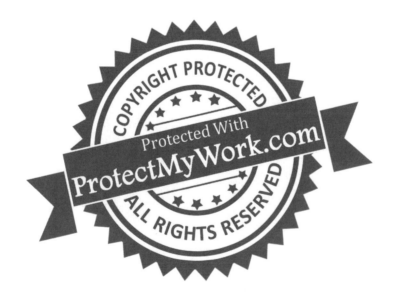

Table of Contents

Introduction

Inside the journey of life, as women gracefully transition into their seventies and beyond, they are met with a series of changes. These changes are not merely external but deeply intertwined with their inner well-being. It's a phase where health takes center stage, and the choices made in terms of nutrition become pivotal.

As a seasoned nutritionist, I have had the privilege of guiding countless women on their path to better health. Among the diverse range of dietary approaches, one stands out as a transformative option for women over 70 – the Ketogenic Diet.

The Ketogenic Diet, often referred to as the "keto diet," is not just a trend; it's a well-researched nutritional strategy that has shown promise in improving various aspects of health. What sets it apart is its unique focus on low-carbohydrate, high-fat consumption. While this might sound counterintuitive, especially in a world that has long demonized fats, it's vital to understand the science behind this dietary choice.

Inside the chapters that follow, we will delve deep into the Ketogenic Diet and its potential benefits for women over 70. We will explore how it can assist in weight management, enhance mental clarity, and potentially contribute to a healthier, more vibrant life.

However, it's crucial to approach this journey with both enthusiasm and caution. While the Ketogenic Diet offers numerous advantages, it's not without its considerations. We will also discuss the potential risks and how to navigate them safely.

Ultimately, this book is designed to be your companion on the path to better health. It's a guide that empowers you with knowledge and practical insights to make informed choices about your nutrition. You'll find a meticulously crafted grocery list to ensure you choose the right products, practical advice for seamless integration of the ketogenic lifestyle, specially tailored keto recipes, a well-structured meal plan, and a fitness regimen designed with the unique needs of women over 70 in mind.

So, let's embark on this journey together, unlocking the potential of the Ketogenic Diet for women over 70, and discovering a path to a healthier and more vibrant you.

Chapter 1: Changes in Body and Health with Age

As we journey through life, our bodies undergo a remarkable series of changes, especially as we reach the milestone of 70 years and beyond. These transformations are not merely superficial; they delve deep into the core of our physiological makeup.

1.1 Exploring Age-Related Physiological Changes

Metabolism and Energy Expenditure. One of the most notable shifts is the slowdown in metabolism. As we age, our bodies tend to burn fewer calories at rest, making it easier to gain weight. Additionally, energy expenditure during physical activities decreases. This change in metabolism can pose challenges for weight management.

Muscle Mass and Strength. Aging often leads to a gradual loss of muscle mass and strength. This condition, known as sarcopenia, can impact mobility and overall functional independence. Maintaining muscle health becomes pivotal in later years.

Bone Health. Aging is closely linked with a decline in bone density, increasing the risk of fractures and osteoporosis. Ensuring adequate calcium intake and weight-bearing exercises is vital to support bone health.

Hormonal Changes. Women experience hormonal fluctuations, especially during menopause. These changes can affect weight distribution, mood, and energy levels. Understanding these hormonal shifts is vital in tailoring dietary choices.

Digestive Changes. The digestive system can become less efficient with age, leading to issues like constipation and decreased nutrient absorption. A well-designed diet can help alleviate these concerns.

Immune System. Aging can weaken the immune system's response, making older individuals more susceptible to infections. Proper nutrition plays a crucial role in supporting immune function.

Chronic Health Conditions. With age, the risk of chronic health conditions like diabetes, heart disease, and hypertension tends to rise. Dietary strategies like the Ketogenic Diet can influence these conditions positively.

Vision and Hearing. With age, vision and hearing can undergo deteriorations. These changes can impact the quality of life and may require interventions like the use of glasses or hearing aids.

Skin Changes. The skin tends to lose its elasticity, becoming thinner and more prone to wrinkles with age. Emphasizing the importance of sun protection and skincare is crucial to preserving skin health in advanced age.

Cardiovascular System. Arteries can harden with age, increasing the risk of heart diseases. Adopting a balanced diet and making regular physical activity a part of your routine can both help assist in keeping your cardiovascular system in good health.

Cognitive Changes. Aging may lead to cognitive changes, including mild memory decline in some individuals. However, it is vital to highlight that the brain has the capacity to adapt and improve through cognitive training.

Lung Function. Lung capacity may decrease with age, making it more important to avoid smoking and maintain an active lifestyle.

1.2 The Role of Ketogenic Diet in Aging Gracefully

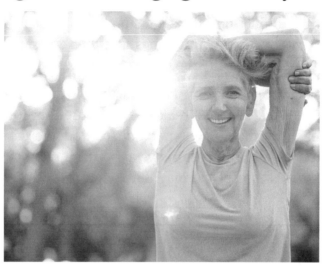

The ketogenic diet, often referred to as the keto diet, has gained substantial attention in recent years for its potential benefits in promoting healthy aging. This dietary approach emphasizes the consumption of high-fat, low-carbohydrate foods, inducing a state of ketosis in the body. The role of the ketogenic diet in aging gracefully encompasses various aspects of physical and cognitive well-being. One of the primary advantages of the keto diet for older adults is its potential to support weight management. With age, maintaining a healthy weight becomes increasingly challenging, and excess weight can lead to various health issues. The keto diet's ability to promote weight loss through the burning of stored fats can be beneficial for older individuals looking to shed extra lbs..

Beyond weight management, the ketogenic diet has shown promise in improving cardiovascular health. By reducing carbohydrate intake and increasing the consumption of heart-healthy fats, it may help in reducing the risk of heart diseases that become more prevalent with age. Cognitive function is another crucial aspect of healthy aging. A few studies suggest that the keto diet may have neuroprotective properties, potentially enhancing brain health and cognitive function in older individuals. While more research is needed in this area, it presents an intriguing avenue for exploration. Moreover, the keto diet's impact on energy levels and vitality in older adults is worth considering. By providing a consistent source of energy through fats, it may help combat fatigue and support an active lifestyle.

In summary, the ketogenic diet holds promise as a dietary strategy for aging gracefully. Its potential benefits in weight management, cardiovascular health, cognitive function, and overall vitality make it a topic of significant interest for those looking to age with grace and maintain a high quality of life.

Chapter 2: The Ketogenic Diet for Women Over 70

2.1 Unraveling the Concept of Ketosis

Ketosis: A Metabolic Shift. Ketosis is at the heart of the ketogenic diet. It's crucial to grasp how this metabolic state works. The metabolic condition known as ketosis occurs when the body switches from using carbs as its main source of energy to using fats instead. This process happens when there is a large reduction in the consumption of carbohydrates, which results in the synthesis of molecules that are known as ketones. Ketones can serve as an alternate source of fuel for several parts of the body, especially the brain.

Why Ketosis Matters. For women over 70, ketosis can hold several benefits. Firstly, it can aid in weight management by encouraging the breakdown of stored fat for energy. This is especially valuable as aging often leads to changes in metabolism and increased fat storage. Secondly, ketosis can help regulate appetite, potentially assisting in portion control and calorie management. Lastly, ketones themselves may have neuroprotective properties that could support cognitive health.

Entering Ketosis. Achieving ketosis requires careful control of macronutrient intake, primarily carbohydrates. Typically, a ketogenic diet limits carb intake to around 20-50 grams per day. This low-carb approach forces the body to deplete its glycogen stores and transition into ketosis. The timeline for entering ketosis varies from person to person but generally takes a couple of days to a week.

Signs of Ketosis. A few common signs of ketosis include increased thirst, changes in breath odor, and reduced appetite. Additionally, many individuals experience an initial drop in weight, mainly due to water loss. Nevertheless, it is essential to keep in mind that people have different sensitivities to ketosis, and therefore not everybody will exhibit the indicators that I have listed.

2.2 Achieving Ketosis Safely for Seniors

For seniors, achieving and maintaining ketosis should be done with care. Here's how:

- ✓ **Dietary Fat Intake:** Seniors should prioritize healthy fats, like avocados, nuts, and olive oil, while avoiding unhealthy trans fats. This shift in fat intake helps the body transition into ketosis.

- ✓ **Protein Moderation:** Protein intake should be moderate. Consuming excessive protein can lead to gluconeogenesis, where protein converts into glucose, potentially disrupting ketosis. It's vital to strike the right balance.

- ✓ **Carbohydrate Restriction:** Limiting carb intake is crucial. Seniors should focus on low-carb vegetables like leafy greens and cruciferous vegetables while avoiding high-carb foods like grains and sugary treats.

- ✓ **Hydration:** Staying well-hydrated is vital, especially for seniors, as they may be more prone to dehydration. Water helps the body process ketones and supports overall health.

- ✓ **Electrolyte Balance:** Ketosis can affect electrolyte levels. Seniors should ensure an adequate intake of sodium, potassium, and magnesium to prevent imbalances.

- ✓ **Medical Supervision:** It's advisable for seniors to consult a healthcare professional before starting a ketogenic diet, especially if they have underlying health conditions or take medications. Medical supervision ensures safety.

- ✓ **Gradual Transition:** Seniors should gradually transition into ketosis, allowing the body to adapt. This approach reduces the risk of adverse effects.

- ✓ **Monitoring Ketone Levels:** It's crucial for beginners in the ketogenic journey, especially women over 70, to have a clear understanding of monitoring ketone levels. Ketone levels indicate whether the body has entered a state of ketosis, which is fundamental for the success of the ketogenic diet. Ketosis is a metabolic state where the body primarily uses ketones, which are produced from fat breakdown, as its energy source instead of carbohydrates. To ensure that ketosis is achieved safely and maintained effectively, regular monitoring is key.

What are Ketone Meters? Ketone meters are user-friendly devices designed to measure the concentration of ketones in the blood. They offer a straightforward way to track your progress on the ketogenic diet. Here's how they work:

- ✓ **Pricking the Finger:** To use a ketone meter, a tiny drop of blood is obtained by pricking the fingertip with a lancet. This process is relatively painless and minimally invasive.

- ✓ **Ketone Strips:** The blood drop is then placed on a specialized ketone strip that is inserted into the meter. These strips contain enzymes that react with the ketones in the blood.

- ✓ **Reading the Results:** Within secs, the meter displays the concentration of ketones in the blood, typically measured in millimoles per liter (mmol/L). This reading provides immediate feedback on whether you are in ketosis.

By regularly using ketone meters, beginners can gain valuable insights into their progress and make informed decisions about their dietary choices. It's an vital tool for ensuring that the ketogenic diet is working effectively and safely, especially for women over 70 who are new to this approach.

2.3 Different Kinds of Keto Diets

Inside the world of ketogenic diets, there are several variations, each with its unique approach and benefits. As you embark on your ketogenic journey, it's vital to understand these different types to choose the one that best suits your needs and preferences. Here, we'll delve into the various kinds of keto diets, explaining each one in detail.

1. Standard Ketogenic Diet (SKD)

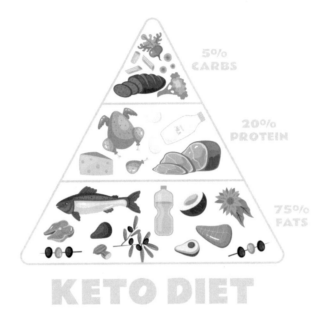

This is the most common and widely practiced form of the ketogenic diet. It involves a high intake of fats, a moderate amount of protein, and a very low intake of carbohydrates. The typical macronutrient ratio is around 70-75% fats, 20-25% protein, and 5-10% carbohydrates. SKD is suitable for those looking to achieve and maintain ketosis effectively. Here are the advantages and disadvantages for women over 70 considering the SDK:

Advantages for Women Over 70

- ✓ **Steady Weight Management:** SKD can aid women over 70 in maintaining a healthy weight. The low carbohydrate intake encourages the body to burn fat for energy, potentially leading to weight loss or weight maintenance, a crucial aspect of senior health.

- ✓ **Blood Sugar Control:** SKD may help regulate blood sugar levels, which is especially beneficial for individuals dealing with age-related insulin resistance or diabetes.

- ✓ **Brain Health:** The high-fat content in SKD provides a rich source of brain-boosting nutrients. For women over 70, this can support cognitive function and potentially reduce the risk of age-related cognitive decline.

Disadvantages for Women Over 70

- ✗ **Potential Nutrient Deficiencies:** SKD can sometimes lead to nutrient deficiencies, especially in vital vitamins and minerals. For women over 70, it's crucial to pay attention to proper micronutrient intake to support overall health.

- ✗ **Digestive Challenges:** A few individuals may experience digestive issues when transitioning to SKD due to the change in fiber intake. This can be more noticeable in older adults. Adequate fiber and hydration are key.

- ✗ **Medication Adjustments:** Women over 70 who are on medications should consult with a healthcare provider when starting SKD, as medication adjustments may be necessary due to the change in metabolic processes.

2. Targeted Ketogenic Diet (TKD)

TKD is designed for individuals who engage in regular physical activities or workouts. It allows for a mildly higher intake of carbohydrates around the time of exercise to provide extra energy. This approach helps athletes or active seniors sustain their performance while staying in ketosis. Here are the advantages and disadvantages for women over 70 considering the TKD:

Advantages for Women Over 70

- ✓ **Enhanced Physical Performance:** TKD's higher carb intake around workouts can provide a boost of energy, making it easier for women over 70 to engage in physical activities without experiencing fatigue.

- ✓ **Muscle Preservation:** For active seniors, TKD can help preserve muscle mass, which is vital for maintaining strength and mobility as one ages.

- ✓ **Improved Recovery:** The additional carbohydrates can aid in post-exercise recovery, reducing the risk of muscle soreness and promoting overall well-being.

Disadvantages for Women Over 70

- ✗ **Precision Required:** TKD requires precise timing of carbohydrate intake around workouts. For some older individuals, this level of precision may be challenging to maintain.

- ✗ **Carb Tolerance:** Older individuals may have varying levels of carb tolerance. In order to identify the proper amount of carb intake, it is necessary to keep a close eye on blood sugar levels and discuss the matter with a qualified medical practitioner.

- ✗ **Individual Variability:** The effectiveness of TKD can vary among individuals. It might not be suitable for everyone, so it's vital to assess whether it aligns with one's fitness goals and body's response.

3. Cyclical Ketogenic Diet (CKD)

CKD involves cycling between periods of strict keto (low-carb) and higher-carb intake. For example, you might follow a strict keto diet for five days, followed by two days of increased carbohydrate consumption. CKD can offer more flexibility and is often preferred by those who find it challenging to stick to a standard keto diet long-term. Here are the advantages and disadvantages for women over 70 considering the CKD:

Advantages for Women Over 70

✓ **Dietary Variety:** CKD allows for a wider variety of foods, including carb-rich options during the carb-loading phase. This variety can be appealing to seniors who may want more diverse meal choices.

✓ **Metabolic Flexibility:** CKD can help older individuals maintain metabolic flexibility, which is crucial for adapting to dietary changes and different energy demands.

✓ **Sustainability:** The cyclical nature of CKD provides a break from strict keto, which some seniors may find challenging to adhere to long-term. This may improve diet adherence for women over 70.

Disadvantages for Women Over 70

✗ **Carb Management:** Properly managing carbohydrate intake during the carb-loading phase is crucial. Older individuals need to carefully monitor their carb consumption to avoid potential blood sugar fluctuations.

✗ **Individual Variability:** CKD's effectiveness can vary from person to person. It's vital for women over 70 to assess how their bodies respond to cycling between keto and carb-loading phases.

✗ **Consultation Required:** Before starting CKD, older individuals should consult with healthcare professionals or nutritionists to ensure it aligns with their specific health goals and dietary needs.

4. High-Protein Ketogenic Diet

This variation maintains the high fat intake but allows for a higher protein intake. It might be suitable for seniors who want to prioritize muscle maintenance or are concerned about getting sufficient protein while following a keto diet.

Advantages for Women Over 70

✓ **Muscle Maintenance:** The High-Protein Ketogenic Diet allows for a higher protein intake, which can be beneficial for seniors looking to prioritize muscle maintenance. It helps prevent muscle loss and supports overall strength.

✓ **Satiety:** Increased protein intake can enhance feelings of fullness and satiety. This can be advantageous for older individuals who may struggle with overeating or cravings.

✓ **Nutrient Density:** A focus on protein-rich foods can provide vital nutrients, especially for seniors who need to meet their dietary requirements more effectively.

Disadvantages for Women Over 70

✗ **Potential for Kidney Strain:** High protein intake may strain the kidneys, especially in individuals with pre-existing kidney issues. Seniors should consult with healthcare professionals to ensure their kidneys can handle the increased protein load.

- × **Digestive Challenges:** Older adults may have digestive sensitivities, and a high-protein diet can sometimes exacerbate these issues. Digestive discomfort may occur in some cases.

- × **Risk of Excess Calories:** While protein is satiating, it's crucial for women over 70 to monitor their calorie intake. Excessive calorie consumption, even from protein, can lead to weight gain.

5. Vegetarian or Vegan Ketogenic Diet

For those who prefer a plant-based approach, vegetarian or vegan keto diets replace animal products with plant-based fats and protein sources while maintaining low carbohydrate intake. It requires careful planning to ensure adequate nutrient intake.

Advantages for Women Over 70

- ✓ **Weight Management:** The Vegetarian or Vegan Ketogenic Diet can support weight management, which is often a concern for seniors. By limiting carbohydrates and focusing on plant-based fats and proteins, it can help with weight control.

- ✓ **Heart Health:** Reducing animal products can be beneficial for heart health. A plant-based approach can lower saturated fat intake, potentially reducing the risk of heart-related issues.

- ✓ **Blood Sugar Control:** For individuals with diabetes or those concerned about blood sugar, a low-carb vegetarian or vegan keto diet can help control blood sugar levels.

Disadvantages for Women Over 70

- × **Nutrient Planning:** A vegetarian or vegan keto diet necessitates careful nutrient planning to ensure seniors receive vital vitamins and minerals. This may require supplementation or a well-balanced selection of plant-based foods.

- × **Protein Intake:** Older adults need to maintain adequate protein intake for muscle and bone health. A plant-based keto diet may require additional attention to protein sources.

- × **Digestive Changes:** As people age, they may experience changes in digestion. A diet rich in plant-based fats and proteins might not be suitable for all seniors and can cause digestive discomfort.

6. Lazy Keto

This version of the keto diet simplifies tracking macronutrients by focusing solely on carbohydrate intake. While it can be more accessible, it might not provide the same precise results as other forms of keto.

Advantages for Women Over 70

- ✓ **Simplicity:** Lazy Keto simplifies the tracking of macronutrients by focusing primarily on carbohydrate intake. This can make it more accessible and less intimidating for seniors who may find detailed tracking challenging.

✓ **Potential Weight Loss:** By reducing carb intake, Lazy Keto can lead to weight loss, which can be beneficial for older adults looking to manage their weight.

Disadvantages for Women Over 70

✗ **Lack of Precision:** Lazy Keto might not provide the same precise results as other forms of the ketogenic diet. Seniors seeking specific health outcomes, like managing blood sugar or addressing medical conditions, might not achieve those goals as effectively.

✗ **Nutrient Balance:** Lazy Keto's simplicity in tracking carbs should not lead to neglecting overall nutrient balance. Seniors must still pay attention to getting vital vitamins and minerals for optimal health.

✗ **Individual Variability:** Seniors have unique nutritional needs, and what works for one individual might not work for an extra. Lazy Keto might not cater to these individual variations effectively.

Understanding these different types of ketogenic diets empowers you to make an informed choice about which one aligns with your goals and lifestyle. Whether you seek strict adherence or flexibility, there's a keto variation that can suit your needs as a beginner, especially if you're a woman over 70 looking to optimize your health through the ketogenic approach.

2.4 Adapting Ketogenic Diet to Suit Older Women

As we explore how to customize the ketogenic diet for older women, it's crucial to understand that dietary needs can vary with age. For women over 70, the ketogenic diet can be highly beneficial, but certain adaptations are necessary to ensure it suits their unique requirements.

✓ **Macronutrient Ratios:** Your body may have different macronutrient needs compared to younger individuals. While the standard keto diet typically consists of approximately 70-75% fat, 20-25% protein, and 5-10% carbohydrates, these ratios might need some modifications for seniors like yourself. A few may find it beneficial to mildly increase protein intake to maintain muscle mass and overall health.

✓ **Micronutrients:** Seniors often require more attention to micronutrients like calcium, vitamin D, and fiber. Incorporating keto-friendly foods rich in these nutrients is vital for your well-being. For example, dairy products, leafy greens, and certain nuts can provide calcium, while fatty fish and egg yolks offer vitamin D.

✓ **Hydration:** Drinking enough water is vital for healthy digestion. Ensure you stay well-hydrated throughout the day to support your digestive system.

✓ **Slowly Increase Fiber Intake:** To prevent digestive discomfort, slowly incorporate fiber-rich foods into your diet. Foods like leafy greens, avocados, and low-carb vegetables can provide the fiber you need.

✓ **Probiotic Foods:** Including probiotic-rich foods like yogurt or kefir in your diet can promote a healthy gut. These foods contain beneficial bacteria that can aid in digestion.

✓ **Chew Your Food:** Take your time when eating and chew your food thoroughly. This simple practice can make digestion more comfortable and efficient.

- ✓ **Monitor Fatty Foods:** While fats are a significant part of the ketogenic diet, be mindful of the types and amounts of fats you consume. A few individuals may experience digestive issues with very high-fat meals, so adjust as needed.

- ✓ **Supplementation:** Depending on your individual needs and medical advice, you may benefit from dietary supplements. Common supplements like calcium, vitamin D, and B vitamins can support your overall well-being.

- ✓ **Portion Control:** Managing portion sizes plays a significant role in weight management and overall health, especially for seniors like yourself. Practice portion control to prevent overeating, which can lead to unwanted weight gain.

- ✓ **Balanced Variety:** Emphasize the importance of a well-balanced, varied diet. Include a range of keto-friendly foods to ensure you receive vital nutrients.

- ✓ **Personal Preferences:** Consider your taste preferences and dietary requirements when planning meals. Customizing your meals can make the diet more enjoyable and sustainable.

- ✓ **Nutrient-Dense Choices:** Opt for nutrient-dense foods rich in vitamins and minerals to support your bone health, heart health, and overall well-being.

- ✓ **Regular Health Check-Ups:** It's vital for you, as a woman over 70 following a ketogenic diet, to schedule regular health check-ups with your healthcare provider. These check-ups help monitor your overall health and ensure that the diet aligns perfectly with your specific needs.

- ✓ **Adjustments Based on Your Responses:** Your response to the ketogenic diet may differ from others. A few may enter ketosis more simply than others, while some may require slight modifications to their macronutrient ratios. Listen to your body and make necessary adjustments based on your individual responses.

Social and Emotional Support

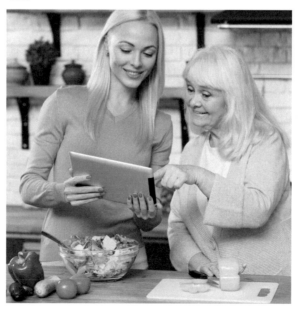

Dietary changes can be challenging, especially as a woman over 70. You might encounter social or emotional obstacles along the way. Here are some practical tips to help you navigate social situations and manage the emotional aspects related to your diet changes:

- ✓ **Communicate Your Goals:** Share your dietary goals with your close friends and family. Let them know why you've chosen the ketogenic diet to support your health. This can foster understanding and support from your loved ones.

- ✓ **Plan Ahead:** When attending social gatherings, plan your meals in advance. If possible, communicate your dietary preferences to the host so they can accommodate your needs.

- ✓ **Stay Positive:** Focus on the positive aspects of your dietary changes, like improved health and vitality. Maintaining a positive mindset can help you stay motivated.

- ✓ **Seek Supportive Communities:** Join online or local communities of individuals following the ketogenic diet. These communities can provide valuable support, tips, and a sense of belonging.

- ✓ **Practice Self-Compassion:** Be kind to yourself throughout your dietary journey. Embrace the occasional indulgence without guilt and remember that progress is a gradual process.

- ✓ **Embrace Mindfulness:** Practice mindfulness during meals. Pay attention to your body's hunger and fullness cues, savor each bite, and enjoy the sensory experience of eating.

Safety Precautions

As a woman over 70, it's vital to be aware of potential side effects or complications related to the ketogenic diet. Here are some safety precautions that you should consider:

- ✓ **Consult with Your Healthcare Provider:** I know I emphasize this point a lot, but it is very important. Before starting any new dietary regimen, consult with your healthcare provider. They can evaluate your specific health needs and advise on whether the ketogenic diet is suitable for you.

- ✓ **Avoid Extreme Restrictions:** While the ketogenic diet can be beneficial, it's important not to overly restrict certain food groups or nutrients. Striking a balanced approach ensures you receive vital nutrients.

- ✓ **Monitor Your Health:** Pay close attention to how your body responds to the diet. If you experience any unusual symptoms or discomfort, consult your healthcare provider promptly.

- ✓ **Medication Adjustments:** If you are taking medications, be aware that the ketogenic diet can sometimes affect their effectiveness. Discuss any necessary adjustments with your healthcare provider.

By following these safety precautions and maintaining open communication with your healthcare provider, you can safely embark on your ketogenic journey. Your health and well-being are our top priorities, and we want to ensure that you make informed choices regarding your diet.

2.5 Balancing Diet and Lifestyle

The ketogenic lifestyle for women over 70 encompasses more than just dietary choices; it embraces a holistic approach to well-being. Let's delve into various facets of your life that play a vital role in achieving balance and success on this journey.

1. Physical Activity. Physical activity should align with your preferences and capabilities. Consider exercises that fit your lifestyle and goals, as they contribute to muscle maintenance, mobility, and overall well-being. Incorporating regular physical activity into your daily routine is vital.

2. Sleep and Stress Management. Quality sleep is the cornerstone of your well-being, especially as a woman over 70. Adequate and restorative sleep plays a pivotal role in maintaining hormonal balance and overall health.

- ✓ **Hormonal Balance:** Sleep directly affects the balance of hormones that regulate various bodily functions. It influences insulin sensitivity, which is vital for stable blood sugar levels, a key component of the ketogenic lifestyle. Proper sleep supports the regulation of appetite hormones, helping you make healthier dietary choices.

- ✓ **Cellular Repair:** During deep sleep phases, your body engages in cellular repair and regeneration. This is crucial for maintaining healthy tissues, organs, and muscles.

- ✓ **Cognitive Function:** Quality sleep enhances cognitive function, memory consolidation, and problem-solving abilities. It contributes to mental clarity and alertness during the day.

Effective stress management is equally vital for women over 70. Chronic stress can have detrimental effects on your health, including elevated cortisol levels, which can hinder ketosis.

- ✓ **Hormone Regulation:** The hormonal balance can be thrown off by chronic stress, which may then give rise to a need for comfort foods that are heavy in carbohydrates. Finding healthy ways to cope with stress might be an important step toward reaching your ketogenic diet objectives.

- ✓ **Heart Health:** Stress management techniques can significantly reduce the risk of cardiovascular issues, which is crucial for maintaining heart health.

- ✓ **Digestive Wellness:** Stress can affect digestion and contribute to digestive discomfort. Managing stress can alleviate these issues.

Customized Sleep Strategies

- ✓ **Sleep Environment:** Creating a comfortable sleep environment is crucial. This may involve optimizing your bedroom for rest by controlling lighting, noise, and temp. to suit your preferences.

- ✓ **Sleep Hygiene:** Establishing good sleep hygiene practices, like maintaining a regular sleep schedule, can improve sleep quality. We will provide guidance on developing a bedtime routine that supports restorative sleep.

- ✓ **Nutrition and Timing:** Your dietary choices and meal timing can impact sleep. We'll explore how to adjust your eating patterns to promote better sleep.

- ✓ **Relaxation Techniques:** Relaxation techniques like deep breathing, progressive muscle relaxation, or gentle yoga can help calm your mind and prepare your body for sleep. We'll guide you through these practices.

3. Social Connections. Maintaining social connections and building a strong support network are vital for overall well-being. Staying connected with loved ones positively influences your health and satisfaction with the ketogenic lifestyle. Social interactions can also impact your dietary choices.

4. Celebrating Progress. Recognizing and celebrating your achievements is vital. Your path to improved health is personal, and acknowledging your successes, no matter how small, can boost your motivation and self-confidence.

2.6 Challenges and Solutions

1. Food Choices at Social Gatherings. When attending social gatherings, it can be challenging to find keto-friendly options. Here are some practical tips for following your diet, even in "difficult" situations:

- ✓ **Lean Proteins:** Look for dishes that feature lean proteins like grilled chicken, turkey, or fish. These options are typically lower in carbohydrates and can be the foundation of your meal.

- ✓ **Vegetables:** Load up on non-starchy vegetables like leafy greens, broccoli, cauliflower, and asparagus. These provide vital nutrients and fiber without a significant carb count.

- ✓ **Healthy Fats:** Seek out sources of healthy fats like avocados, olive oil, and nuts. These fats can help you feel satiated and provide vital nutrients.

- ✓ **Avoid Sugary Sauces:** Be cautious of sauces and dressings, as they often contain hidden sugars and carbohydrates. Opt for options with minimal sugar content or request sauces on the side.

- ✓ **Beverage Choices:** Choose water, unsweetened tea, or sparkling water as your beverages to avoid unnecessary sugar and carbs from sodas and sugary drinks.

2. Effective Communication. Communication is vital in ensuring you can enjoy social events while sticking to your dietary goals:

- ✓ **Express Your Preferences:** Don't hesitate to inform hosts or friends about your dietary preferences and restrictions. Most people are accommodating and will appreciate your honesty.

- ✓ **Offer to Contribute:** When attending potluck-style gatherings, offer to bring a keto-friendly dish to share. This guarantees that you have an option you can enjoy while also introducing others to delicious keto recipes.

- ✓ **Ask Questions:** If you're unsure about the components in a dish, don't be afraid to ask the host for details. It's better to be informed about what you're eating.

- ✓ **Special Requests:** Don't hesitate to make special requests when dining out.

3. Strategic Meal Planning. Planning ahead is a valuable tool for staying on track with your ketogenic diet during social gatherings:

- ✓ **Plan Your Dish:** If possible, coordinate with the host to plan a keto-friendly dish that you can enjoy. This ensures you have a satisfying option available.

- ✓ **Prepare in Advance:** Consider preparing keto-friendly snacks or appetizers in advance, so you always have something suitable to nibble on.

- ✓ **BYO:** If necessary, bring your own keto-friendly dish to social events. This guarantees you'll have a meal that aligns with your dietary needs.

- ✓ **Eat Beforehand:** If you anticipate limited keto options, eat a small keto-friendly meal or snack before the gathering to reduce the temptation to indulge in non-keto foods.

4. Managing Cravings. Understanding true hunger cues is crucial for distinguishing between genuine hunger and cravings. Genuine hunger comes with distinct physical sensations and signals from your body. These cues include:

- ✓ **Stomach Sensations:** True hunger often manifests as a sensation of emptiness or a gentle rumbling in the stomach. This physical signal indicates that your body needs nourishment.

- ✓ **Physical Weakness:** Genuine hunger can lead to feelings of weakness or low energy levels. Your body signals the need for fuel to regain vitality.

- ✓ **Consistent Timing:** True hunger tends to follow a consistent schedule, aligning with your typical meal times. It builds gradually and becomes more noticeable as time since your last meal or snack increases.

- ✓ **Lack of Food Thoughts:** When you're genuinely hungry, you may think about food in a practical, non-obsessive way. The thought of eating is driven by a physical need rather than an emotional craving.

Paying attention to these physical signals can help you make mindful choices and respond to your body's actual nutritional needs. Emotions often lead to cravings, which can mimic feelings of hunger. Recognizing emotional triggers is vital to differentiate between emotional desires and genuine hunger. Common emotional triggers include:

- ✓ **Stress:** Stress can create a desire for comforting foods as a way to cope with emotional tension. This can lead to cravings for specific comfort foods.

- ✓ **Boredom:** When you're bored, food can become a source of entertainment or distraction. This may lead to cravings even when you're not truly hungry.

- ✓ **Sadness or Loneliness:** Emotional states like sadness or loneliness can trigger cravings for foods that provide a temporary sense of comfort or pleasure.
- ✓ **Habitual Eating:** A fewtimes, you may feel like eating simply out of habit, not because you're hungry. These habitual eating patterns can lead to cravings that are not based on genuine hunger.

By practicing mindful eating, you can enhance your ability to differentiate between true hunger and cravings. Mindful eating is a practice that can help you differentiate between genuine hunger and cravings. It involves:

- ✓ **Paying Attention:** Being fully present during meals and snacks, focusing on the sensory experience of eating, including taste, texture, and aroma.
- ✓ **Engage Your Senses:** Pay attention to the colors, smells, and textures of your food. It enhances the experience.
- ✓ **Chew Thoroughly:** Chew your food slowly and thoroughly. It allows your body to signal when it's full.
- ✓ **Pause Between Bites:** Put your utensils down between bites. This slows the pace of your meal.
- ✓ **Appreciate Your Food:** Be grateful for the nourishment your meal provides.
- ✓ **Listening to Your Body:** Tuning into your body's hunger and fullness cues. Before eating, ask yourself if you're truly hungry, and after eating, assess your level of fullness.
- ✓ **Eating with Awareness:** Avoiding distractions while eating, like watching TV or scrolling through your phone. This allows you to savor each bite and be more in tune with your body's signals.
- ✓ **Non-Judgmental Observation:** Approaching your eating habits with curiosity and without self-criticism. Mindful eating is about developing a compassionate and non-judgmental relationship with food.
- ✓ **Savoring Each Bite**: As we age, our sense of taste can change. Mindful eating encourages savoring each bite, making meals more enjoyable.
- ✓ **Portion Control:** Mindful eating helps with portion control, preventing overeating, which is vital when following a ketogenic diet.
- ✓ **Emotional Well-Being:** Mindful eating fosters a positive relationship with food, reducing emotional eating tendencies.

5. Smart Snacking. Having keto-friendly snacks readily available is vital when cravings strike. Here's a detailed look at handling snacking:

- ✓ **Nuts:** Almonds, walnuts, and macadamia nuts are excellent choices for healthy fats and a satisfying crunch.
- ✓ **Seeds:** Chia seeds, flaxseeds, and pumpkin seeds provide fiber and nutrients.
- ✓ **Cheese:** Cheese sticks or cubes are rich in both flavor and healthy fats.

✓ **Vegetables with Dip:** Crisp, low-carb vegetables like cucumber, celery, and bell peppers paired with keto-friendly dips.

Of course, portion control matters when snacking. Properly portioned snacks serve several purposes, including:

✓ **Managing Calorie Intake:** By controlling the quantity of snacks you consume, you can better manage your overall calorie intake. This is vital for weight management and staying in a calorie deficit if your goal is weight loss.

✓ **Staying within Daily Carb Limits:** For a ketogenic diet, it's vital to monitor your carbohydrate intake closely. Proper portion control ensures that you don't exceed your daily carb limit while enjoying snacks.

✓ **Curbing Cravings:** Snacking in moderation can help curb cravings without derailing your diet. By eating the right portion size, you satisfy your hunger without overindulging.

Here there are some practical strategies for effective portion control when snacking:

✓ **Measuring Portions:** Using measuring teacups or a food scale to measure out your snacks can be an eye-opening experience. It helps you become aware of what an appropriate portion looks like.

✓ **Pre-Portioning:** Pre-portioning snacks into individual servings can prevent mindless eating. It's especially helpful for snacks like nuts or seeds, where it's easy to lose track of how much you've eaten.

✓ **Snack Packaging:** Choosing snacks that come in single-presenting packages can simplify portion control. This eliminates the need for measuring and helps you avoid overindulging.

6. Occasional Treats. How to incorporate occasional treats into your ketogenic lifestyle without compromising your progress? Making informed choices when selecting treats is crucial. You can opt for dark chocolate with a higher cocoa content as it tends to be lower in carbohydrates compared to milk chocolate. Additionally, consider sugar-free or keto-friendly desserts as suitable alternatives to traditional high-carb treats. As I have already said before, practicing moderation is key to mindful indulgence. On a ketogenic diet, you have a specific daily limit for carbohydrate consumption to maintain ketosis. Consuming too many carbs, even from keto-friendly sources, can potentially disrupt ketosis and hinder your progress. Be mindful of how the occasional treat fits into your daily carb budget. Moreover, it's vital to find a balance between enjoying occasional treats and staying true to your keto goals. Remember that these treats should enhance your overall keto experience rather than become the primary focus of your diet. They are a part of a sustainable approach to keto, allowing you to savor special moments without compromising your long-term health objectives. By practicing moderation and staying within your daily carb limits, you can relish occasional treats while ensuring that your ketogenic journey remains on track. This balanced approach not only supports your dietary success but also promotes a healthier relationship with food and helps you achieve and maintain your desired health outcomes.

Chapter 3: Benefits and Risks of the Ketogenic Diet

3.1 Discovering the Pros of Ketogenic Diet for Older Women

In this chapter, we'll explore the many advantages that the ketogenic diet can offer to women over the age of 70. It's important to remember that every individual's journey with the ketogenic diet is unique, and while it may present certain challenges, it also brings forth numerous benefits, especially for older women.

1. Weight Management and Fat Loss. Weight management becomes increasingly vital as we age, and the ketogenic diet has shown promise in this area. By reducing carbohydrate intake and emphasizing healthy fats and lean proteins, the diet can promote fat loss while preserving muscle mass. For women over 70, this can be especially beneficial in maintaining a healthy body composition and supporting overall well-being.

2. Improved Metabolic Health. Cognitive health is a priority for women as they age. The ketogenic diet has gained attention for its potential to support brain function. By providing the brain with ketones as an alternative energy source, it may offer neuroprotective benefits. A few studies suggest that the diet may help enhance memory, cognitive performance, and reduce the risk of neurodegenerative diseases. One noteworthy nutrient found in the ketogenic diet that plays a pivotal role in supporting brain health is docosahexaenoic acid (DHA). DHA is a remarkable omega-3 fatty acid, predominantly abundant in fatty fish like salmon and mackerel. DHA's significance lies in its ability to maintain the integrity of brain cell membranes. These membranes are the guardians of your brain cells, and DHA acts as their protector, ensuring they remain strong and resilient. Moreover, DHA supports communication between brain cells, facilitating the seamless exchange of information in this intricate network.

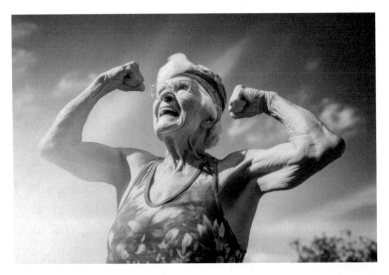

3. Increased Energy Levels. Sustaining energy levels becomes more challenging with age, but the ketogenic diet's reliance on fat for energy can lead to sustained and stable energy throughout the day. Many women over 70 report feeling more energetic and alert after adopting the diet.

4. Better Heart Health. The ketogenic diet can promote heart health by reducing triglyceride levels and increasing levels of high-density lipoprotein (HDL) cholesterol. These changes are linked with a lower risk of cardiovascular disease. Older women who are concerned about heart health can find reassurance in these potential benefits.

5. Appetite Regulation. One of the remarkable aspects of the ketogenic diet is its ability to stabilize blood sugar levels, providing a steady source of energy throughout the day. This stability in blood sugar levels is key to reducing hunger spikes and enhancing appetite control. When you consume carbohydrates in your diet, they can lead to rapid spikes and crashes in blood sugar levels. These fluctuations often result in cravings and overeating, which can be challenging to manage, especially as we age. However, the ketogenic diet takes a different approach. By emphasizing low-carb, high-fat foods, it promotes a consistent and steady blood sugar level. The benefit of this stability is twofold. Firstly, it helps prevent sudden cravings that often derail dietary goals. Secondly, it fosters a feeling of fullness, which can be especially advantageous for older women. This improved appetite control can make it significantly easier to manage food intake and adhere to your dietary objectives.

6. Enhanced Bone Health. For older women, maintaining strong bones is vital. While some concerns have been raised about the diet's impact on bone health, it's possible to follow a ketogenic diet that comprises foods rich in calcium and vitamin D. These nutrients play a vital role in bone strength and overall bone health. Leafy green vegetables like kale and spinach are excellent natural sources of calcium that align perfectly with the principles of the ketogenic diet. These greens can be simply integrated into your keto meals, ensuring you receive the calcium your bones require. Furthermore, low-carb dairy products, like Greek yogurt and cheese, not only provide calcium but also contribute to your vitamin D intake. Vitamin D is crucial for calcium absorption and bone health. Ensuring these foods are part of your dietary plan can help you maintain strong and resilient bones, which is especially pertinent for older women who wish to safeguard their bone health throughout the aging process.

7. Stable Blood Pressure. The ketogenic diet may help lower blood pressure in some individuals, which is vital for maintaining cardiovascular health. However, it's crucial to monitor blood pressure regularly, especially if you are taking medications, and consult with a healthcare professional.

3.2 Navigating Potential Risks and Challenges

As we explore the ketogenic diet and its potential benefits for women over 70, it's crucial to also acknowledge and address potential risks and challenges linked with this dietary approach. While the keto diet offers many advantages, it's vital to make informed choices and be aware of possible difficulties that may arise during your journey.

1. Nutrient Intake. One challenge of the ketogenic diet is ensuring that you receive an adequate intake of vital nutrients. The diet restricts carbohydrates, which are a primary source of many vitamins and minerals. To mitigate this risk, it's vital to focus on a well-balanced keto diet that incorporates a variety of non-starchy vegetables, lean proteins, and healthy fats.

Additionally, consider taking supplements to cover any potential nutrient gaps, especially important for women over 70 who may have specific nutritional needs.

2. Digestive Issues. A few individuals may experience digestive discomfort when transitioning to a keto diet. This can include constipation, diarrhea, or other gastrointestinal disturbances. To address these challenges, it's advisable to gradually increase your fiber intake from keto-friendly sources like leafy greens, nuts, and seeds. Staying hydrated and incorporating fermented foods can also promote digestive health.

3. Potential Side Effects. The keto diet can sometimes lead to side effects known as the "keto flu," which may include fatigue, headache, and nausea during the initial stages of ketosis. While these symptoms are typically temporary, it's vital to stay well-hydrated, consume adequate electrolytes, and get plenty of rest to ease the transition.

4. Monitoring Ketosis. Achieving and maintaining ketosis, the metabolic state where your body burns fat for fuel, is a primary goal of the ketogenic diet. However, it can be challenging to monitor your ketone levels accurately. Consider using ketone testing strips or blood ketone meters to track your progress and ensure you are in a state of ketosis.

5. Individual Variability. Keep in mind that individual responses to the ketogenic diet can vary. What works well for one person might not have the same effect on another. Therefore, it's vital to listen to your body, pay attention to how you feel, and make adjustments to your dietary plan as needed.

6. Medical Considerations. I have already said this before, but some medications may interact with the ketogenic diet and have different effects. It's vital to consult with a healthcare provider to monitor medication effectiveness and make any necessary adjustments while following the diet. Certain medical conditions may require modified versions of the diet or close monitoring.

7. Bone Health. Older women may be more susceptible to bone health issues like osteoporosis. The ketogenic diet can potentially affect calcium and magnesium levels in the body. It's important to ensure you're getting an adequate amount of these nutrients through foods or supplements if necessary to support bone health.

8. Dehydration. The ketogenic diet can have a diuretic effect, meaning it may increase fluid loss through urine. Older women may already be more susceptible to dehydration, so it's crucial to maintain proper hydration levels while on the diet. To prevent dehydration while following the ketogenic diet, it's vital to have a clear understanding of your daily water intake needs. For women over 70, who may be more susceptible to dehydration, a general guideline is to aim for almost 8 to 10 teacups of water per day. This translates to approximately 64 to 80 oz. of water, though individual requirements may vary based on factors like climate, activity level, and overall health. Incorporate regular water intake into your daily routine and be attentive to your body's signals for thirst. Dehydration can lead to various side effects, which can be especially challenging for individuals on a keto diet. By prioritizing adequate hydration, you can reduce the risk of these side effects and ensure your body functions optimally throughout your ketogenic journey.

9. Long-Term Sustainability. Maintaining a ketogenic diet over the long term can be challenging for some individuals. Older women should consider the sustainability of the diet and whether it aligns with their lifestyle and preferences.

3.3 Managing Ketogenic Diet Side Effects

How to manage potential side effects? Here there are some tips:

✓ A few individuals may experience flu-like symptoms when initially transitioning into ketosis. Combat this by staying hydrated, replenishing electrolytes, and ensuring adequate rest.

✓ A few individuals may experience constipation on a ketogenic diet. Increase your fiber intake through low-carb vegetables and consider adding a fiber supplement if needed.

✓ Muscle cramps can result from electrolyte imbalances. Include magnesium-rich foods or supplements to help prevent cramping.

✓ Ketosis may lead to increased fluid loss through urine. Drink water consistently to stay hydrated, and consider adding an electrolyte supplement if needed.

✓ A few individuals may experience increased hunger or cravings initially. Focus on satisfying, keto-friendly foods and practice mindful eating to manage these urges.

✓ While your body adapts to ketosis, you might notice changes in energy levels. Ensure you're consuming enough calories and give your body time to adjust.

✓ Be mindful of potential nutrient deficiencies, especially calcium and potassium. Consult with a healthcare provider to determine if supplementation is necessary.

✓ Monitor your cholesterol levels regularly, as a ketogenic diet can affect cholesterol markers. Consult with your healthcare provider to assess and manage any changes.

✓ Navigating social gatherings and dining out can be challenging. Plan ahead, communicate your dietary preferences, and be prepared with keto-friendly options to stay on track.

3.3 Encouraging Seniors to Embark on Their Ketogenic Journey

Embarking on a ketogenic journey as a senior, especially as a woman over 70, can be a rewarding and transformative experience. It's vital to approach this lifestyle change with confidence and enthusiasm. Here's a heartfelt guide to inspire and support you on your ketogenic journey:

✓ **Believe in Your Strength:** Understand that age is just a number, and you possess the strength and resilience to make positive changes in your life. Embrace the idea that it's never too late to prioritize your health and well-being.

✓ **Start Slow and Steady:** Begin your ketogenic journey gradually. Make small dietary adjustments and allow your body to adapt to this new way of eating. Progress at your own pace, focusing on sustainability over quick results.

✓ **Seek Support and Consult with Professionals**

- ✓ **Variety in Meal Preparation:** Keep your ketogenic journey exciting and fresh by exploring a wide range of keto-friendly recipes and components. Don't be afraid to experiment with different flavors and textures. Variety not only adds excitement to your meals but also ensures you get a diverse array of nutrients.

- ✓ **Find Pleasure in Keto Cooking:** Cooking can be a delightful and creative experience. Embrace the joy of keto cooking by trying new recipes and discovering inventive ways to prepare your favorite dishes. Finding pleasure in the preparation process can make the ketogenic diet an enjoyable part of your daily routine.

- ✓ **Educate Yourself:** Knowledge is a powerful tool. Take the time to educate yourself about the ketogenic diet, its principles, and its potential benefits. Understanding the "why" behind this lifestyle can reinforce your commitment.

- ✓ **Celebrate Milestone**

- ✓ **Embrace a Positive Mindset:** Cultivate a positive and compassionate mindset towards yourself. Be patient and understanding, knowing that every step forward is a step toward better health.

- ✓ **Positive Relationship with Food:** Foster a positive and healthy relationship with food. Recognize that the ketogenic diet is not about deprivation but about nourishing your body with wholesome, satisfying foods. By maintaining a positive attitude towards food, you can sustain this way of eating in the long run.

- ✓ **Stay Curious:** Keep a curious spirit and stay open to new experiences and knowledge. The ketogenic journey can be a wonderful opportunity for personal growth and exploration.

- ✓ **Enjoy the Journey:** Lastly, remember that your ketogenic journey is not just about reaching a destination; it's about the experience along the way. Savor the moments, enjoy delicious meals, and relish the newfound vitality it brings to your life.

Embarking on a ketogenic journey as a senior is a remarkable step towards improved health and well-being. Approach it with determination, self-compassion, and a sense of adventure. Your journey is uniquely yours, and every day is an opportunity to thrive on this path to wellness.

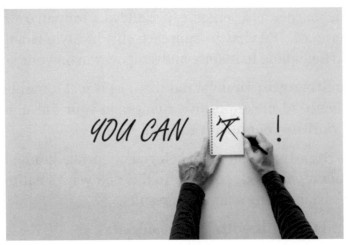

Chapter 4: KETO GROCERY LIST

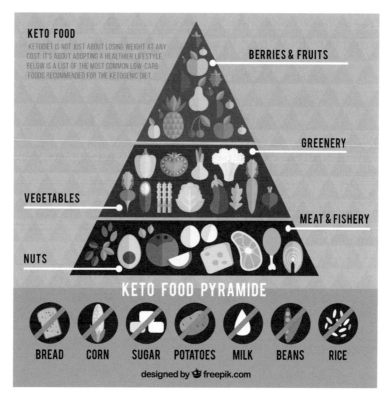

4.1 Foods to Buy for Your Ketogenic Journey

As you embark on your ketogenic journey, it's vital to stock your kitchen with the right foods to support your new way of eating. Here, we'll explore the foods you should consider adding to your grocery list as a woman over 70 following the ketogenic diet.

1. Healthy Fats

✓ Avocados

✓ Coconut oil

✓ Olive oil

✓ Grass-fed butter

Healthy fats are the cornerstone of the ketogenic diet. These fats provide vital nutrients and are a primary source of energy on keto.

2. Protein Sources

✓ Skinless poultry (chicken, turkey)

✓ Lean cuts of beef or pork

✓ Fatty fish (salmon, mackerel)

✓ Eggs (organic and pasture-raised)

Lean proteins are vital for muscle maintenance and overall health. Opt for organic and pasture-raised options when possible.

3. Low-Carb Vegetables

✓ Leafy greens (spinach, kale, arugula)

✓ Broccoli

✓ Cauliflower

✓ Zucchini

- ✓ Asparagus
- ✓ Bell peppers
- ✓ Cucumbers

Non-starchy vegetables are rich in vitamins, minerals, and fiber while being low in carbs. These vegetables are versatile and can be utilized in various keto-friendly recipes.

4. Nuts and Seeds

- ✓ Almonds
- ✓ Walnuts
- ✓ Chia seeds
- ✓ Flaxseeds

Nuts and seeds are excellent sources of healthy fats and provide a satisfying crunch.

5. Dairy Products

- ✓ Cheese (various types like cheddar, mozzarella, and cream cheese)
- ✓ Full-fat yogurt (unsweetened)
- ✓ Heavy cream

If you tolerate dairy, include these items. These dairy products can include flavor and richness to your keto meals.

6. Berries

- ✓ Strawberries
- ✓ Blueberries
- ✓ Raspberries

While fruits are generally limited on keto due to their sugar content, berries are lower in carbs and can be enjoyed in moderation.

7. Herbs and Spices

- ✓ Garlic
- ✓ Basil
- ✓ Oregano
- ✓ Cinnamon

Enhance the flavor of your meals with herbs and spices. They will include depth and variety to your dishes.

8. Keto-Friendly Sweeteners

- ✓ Stevia
- ✓ Erythritol
- ✓ Monk fruit sweetener

If you have a sweet tooth, look for keto-friendly sweeteners. These can be utilized as sugar substitutes in keto-friendly desserts.

9. Canned and Jarred Items

- ✓ Canned tuna or salmon
- ✓ Olives
- ✓ Pickles

These canned and jarred products are keto-friendly. Check labels for added sugars and choose options with no or minimal carbs.

10. Keto-Friendly Snacks

- ✓ Pork rinds
- ✓ Beef jerky
- ✓ Sugar-free dark chocolate

Keep keto snacks on hand for when cravings strike. These snacks can help you stay on track while satisfying your munchies.

11. Keto-Friendly Drinks

✓ **Water:** Water is vital for maintaining hydration and overall health. It's the best choice for a keto-friendly beverage.

✓ **Unsweetened Tea:** Teas like green tea, black tea, and herbal tea are excellent options. Make sure not to include sugar or high-carb sweeteners.

✓ **Black Coffee:** Black coffee is a low-calorie and low-carb beverage, but avoid adding sugar. You can include cream or butter if you follow a variant of the ketogenic diet known as "bulletproof coffee."

✓ **Natural Sparkling Water:** Sugar-free sparkling water is a refreshing and keto-friendly choice.

✓ **Bone Broth:** Bone broth is rich in nutrients and can be an excellent beverage to support hydration and electrolyte balance during a ketogenic diet.

✓ **Erythritol or Stevia-Based Drinks:** A few beverages sweetened with erythritol or stevia can be keto-friendly options. Just check the labels to ensure they don't contain high-carb components.

✓ **Coconut Water (in moderation):** While coconut water contains some carbohydrates, it can be consumed in moderation if it fits within your daily carb limit. It's a natural source of electrolytes.

✓ **Keto Smoothies (homemade):** You can make keto-friendly smoothies using components like unsweetened almond milk, low-carb berries, spinach, and a keto-friendly sweetener like stevia or erythritol.

Remember to read labels and check for hidden sugars or high-carb additives in any packaged drinks.

4.2 Supplements

Depending on your specific dietary needs, you may consider adding supplements like electrolytes or vitamins to support your health. Consult with a healthcare professional for personalized recommendations.

✓ **Multivitamin and Mineral Supplement:** To ensure you meet your daily nutrient needs.

✓ **Vitamin D:** Especially important for older adults to support bone health and overall wellbeing.

✓ **Omega-3 Fatty Acids:** Fish oil supplements can help with joint health and inflammation.

✓ **Electrolyte Supplements:** Potassium, magnesium, and sodium supplements can help maintain electrolyte balance on a ketogenic diet.

✓ **Collagen Powder:** Supports skin, hair, and joint health.

✓ **Fiber Supplement (if needed):** Psyllium husk or other keto-friendly fiber supplements to support digestive health.

✓ **Calcium and Magnesium:** Calcium is important for bone health, especially in older women, while magnesium supports heart and muscle health.

✓ **Vitamin B12:** Older adults may have an increased need for vitamin B12, which is vital for nerve and cognitive health.

✓ **Probiotics:** Probiotics can help support digestive and immune health.

✓ **Coenzyme Q10 (CoQ10):** This antioxidant may help support heart health and energy production.

4.3 Foods To Avoid

1. Sugar

- ✗ White sugar
- ✗ Brown sugar
- ✗ Honey
- ✗ Maple syrup
- ✗ Agave nectar

Avoid all forms of sugar.

2. Grains

- ✗ Wheat
- ✗ Rice
- ✗ Oats
- ✗ Corn

Eliminate grains, as they are high in carbohydrates.

3. Starchy Vegetables

- ✗ Potatoes
- ✗ Sweet potatoes
- ✗ Peas

Limit starchy vegetables, as they contain more carbs.

4. Processed Foods

- ✗ Chips
- ✗ Cookies
- ✗ Sugary snacks

5. High-Carb Fruits

- ✗ Bananas
- ✗ Grapes
- ✗ Mangoes

6. Legumes

- ✗ Beans
- ✗ Lentils
- ✗ Chickpeas

7. Low-Fat Dairy

- ✗ Low-fat or fat-free dairy products

Opt for full-fat dairy options instead of low-fat or fat-free versions.

8. Sugary Beverages

- ✗ Soda
- ✗ Fruit juices
- ✗ Sweetened teas

9. Trans Fats

- ✗ Foods containing trans fats, often found in fried and processed foods

10. Alcohol

Limit alcohol consumption, as it can hinder ketosis and include unnecessary carbs.

11. Artificial Sweeteners

- ✗ Aspartame
- ✗ Sucralose
- ✗ Saccharin

12. Processed Meats

- ✗ Sausages with added sugar or fillers
- ✗ Processed deli meats with added sugars

13. High-Carb Sauces and Condiments

- ✗ Ketchup (often high in sugar)
- ✗ Barbecue sauce (often high in sugar)
- ✗ Salad dressings with added sugars

14. High-Sugar Snack Bars:

- ✗ Snack bars labeled as "healthy" but containing high sugar content

15. Baked Goods

- ✗ Cakes
- ✗ Pastries
- ✗ Cookies
- ✗ Breads (non-keto varieties)

16. High-Carb Nuts and Seeds

- ✗ Cashews (higher in carbs compared to other nuts)
- ✗ Peanuts (legumes, not nuts)

Chapter 5: Exercise and Fitness for Women Over 70 on a Ketogenic Diet

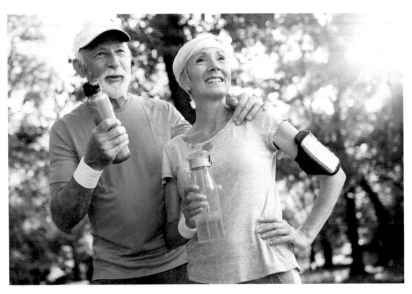

5.1 Embracing Physical Activity for Healthy Aging

Physical activity plays a vital role in promoting healthy aging for women over the age of 70 who are following a ketogenic diet. Engaging in regular exercise is not only compatible with the ketogenic lifestyle but also synergizes with its benefits, contributing to your overall well-being.

1. Strength and Muscle Maintenance: As we age, maintaining muscle mass and strength becomes increasingly crucial for everyday activities and independence. Incorporating resistance training into your fitness routine can help you build and preserve muscle. Activities like lifting weights or using resistance bands can be adapted to your fitness level and provide substantial benefits.

2. Cardiovascular Health: Cardiovascular exercise is vital for a healthy heart and circulatory system. Activities like brisk walking, swimming, or cycling can improve cardiovascular fitness, reduce the risk of heart disease, and enhance endurance. Even low-impact exercises can significantly contribute to heart health.

3. Flexibility and Mobility: Aging can bring about changes in flexibility and joint mobility. Including stretching exercises in your regimen can enhance your range of motion, prevent stiffness, and reduce the risk of injury. Incorporate gentle yoga or stretching routines to maintain flexibility.

4. Balance and Coordination: Balance and coordination are fundamental for preventing falls and maintaining stability. Engage in balance exercises, like standing on one leg or Tai Chi, to improve your equilibrium and reduce the risk of accidents.

5. Adaptation to Keto Fuel: As you exercise on a ketogenic diet, your body becomes efficient at using ketones for energy. This adaptation can lead to improved endurance during workouts.

It's vital to stay adequately hydrated and maintain your electrolyte balance during exercise to support your body's performance.

6. Consistency is Key: Consistency in your exercise routine is vital for reaping the benefits of physical activity. Aim for a regular schedule that comprises a mix of strength, cardiovascular, flexibility, and balance exercises. Staying active consistently can lead to improved overall health and vitality.

Benefits of Physical Activity for Women Over 70

Engaging in regular physical activity offers numerous advantages for women over the age of 70. These benefits extend beyond physical health and encompass various aspects of well-being. Here, we explore the positive impacts of staying active:

- ✓ **Enhanced Physical Health:** Regular exercise contributes to improved cardiovascular health, reduced risk of chronic diseases like heart disease and diabetes, and enhanced overall physical fitness. It helps maintain a healthy weight, which is vital for mobility and joint health.

- ✓ **Increased Energy Levels:** Contrary to the belief that exercise depletes energy, staying active can boost your energy levels. Physical activity enhances the circulation of oxygen and nutrients throughout your body, leaving you feeling more energized and alert.

- ✓ **Improved Mental Well-Being:** Exercise has a profound effect on mental health. It can reduce symptoms of anxiety and depression, enhance mood, and promote feelings of happiness and relaxation. Engaging in physical activity can also improve cognitive function and memory.

- ✓ **Enhanced Quality of Life:** An active lifestyle can enhance your overall quality of life. It enables you to engage in daily activities with greater ease, maintain independence, and pursue hobbies and interests. Staying physically active can contribute to a more fulfilling and enjoyable life in your senior years.

- ✓ **Social Interaction:** Participating in group activities or classes can provide opportunities for social interaction and community engagement. Building connections with others who share your interests can combat feelings of isolation and loneliness.

- ✓ **Better Sleep:** Exercise can promote better sleep patterns, helping you fall asleep faster and enjoy more restorative sleep. Adequate rest is crucial for overall well-being, and physical activity can play a significant role in achieving it.

5.2 Precautions to Take for Physical Activity for Women Over 70

While physical activity offers numerous benefits, it's vital to take certain precautions, especially as a woman over 70, to ensure safe and enjoyable exercise experiences. Here are some considerations:

- ✓ **Consult with a Healthcare Provider:** Before beginning a new exercise regimen, consult with your healthcare provider. They can assess your current health status, provide recommendations, and help you identify any potential limitations or concerns.

- ✓ **Choose Appropriate Activities:** Select physical activities that are suitable for your fitness level and individual needs. Low-impact exercises like walking, swimming, or gentle yoga can be gentle on the joints while still providing benefits.

- ✓ **Warm-Up and Cool Down:** Always include warm-up and cool-down periods in your exercise routine. These phases are crucial for preparing your body for activity and reducing the risk of injury. Stretching can improve flexibility and prevent muscle strain.

- ✓ **Stay Hydrated:** Dehydration can be a concern during physical activity, so ensure you stay adequately hydrated. Drink water before, during, and after your workouts, especially in warm weather.

- ✓ **Listen to Your Body:** Pay attention to your body's signals during exercise. If you experience pain, dizziness, shortness of breath, or any unusual symptoms, stop the activity instantly and seek medical attention if necessary. It's crucial to exercise at a pace that feels comfortable for you.

- ✓ **Balance and Coordination:** Exercises that focus on balance and coordination are vital for preventing falls and maintaining stability. Consider including balance-specific workouts in your routine.

- ✓ **Rest and Recovery:** Adequate rest and recovery are vital, especially as you age. Allow your body time to recover between workouts, and don't overexert yourself. Listen to your body's need for rest.

- ✓ **Nutritional Adequacy:** Ensure that your ketogenic diet provides sufficient nutrients to support physical activity. Monitor your intake of vital nutrients like protein, vitamins, and minerals, which are crucial for muscle health and overall well-being. If needed, consult with a healthcare provider or a registered dietitian to address any potential nutrient deficiencies.

- ✓ **Gradual Progression:** Start your exercise routine gradually and progress at your own pace. Avoid overexertion and sudden, intense workouts, especially if you are new to exercise or have been sedentary for a while. Slowly increase the intensity and duration of your workouts as your fitness level improves.

- ✓ **Proper Footwear:** Choose appropriate footwear that provides support and comfort for your chosen physical activities. Ill-fitting or unsuitable shoes can lead to discomfort and increase the risk of injuries, especially when engaging in weight-bearing exercises.

- ✓ **Joint Care**: Pay attention to joint health, as it becomes increasingly important with age. Consider low-impact exercises like swimming or cycling to minimize stress on joints. If you experience joint pain, consult with a healthcare provider for guidance and potential modifications to your exercise routine.

- ✓ **Regular Monitoring:** Keep a record of your exercise activities and monitor your progress over time. Regular tracking can help you stay motivated and identify any changes in your fitness level. It can also provide valuable information to share with your healthcare provider.

- ✓ **Recovery Strategies:** Implement effective recovery strategies to minimize muscle soreness and optimize recovery between workouts. Techniques like foam rolling, gentle stretching, and adequate rest can aid in recovery and reduce the risk of overuse injuries.

- ✓ **Safety Measures:** Ensure that you exercise in a safe environment. Use proper equipment, maintain good posture, and be aware of your surroundings to prevent accidents. If you exercise outdoors, consider factors like weather conditions and visibility.

- ✓ **Consultation:** Continue to maintain open communication with your healthcare provider throughout your exercise journey. Discuss any concerns, changes in your health, or modifications needed in your exercise routine.

- ✓ **Social Support:** Engage in physical activities with others whenever possible. Exercising in a group or with friends can provide motivation, social interaction, and a sense of community, making the experience more enjoyable and sustainable.

- ✓ **Adaptation:** Be adaptable and willing to modify your exercise routine as needed. Aging may come with certain physical changes, and it's vital to adjust your activities to accommodate these changes while still staying active and engaged.

Remember that safety and individualization are key when combining a ketogenic diet with physical activity in your senior years. Always prioritize your health and well-being, and consult with healthcare professionals or fitness experts as needed to create a tailored and safe exercise plan.

5.3 21-Day Exercise Plan For Women (Compatible with Keto Lifestyle)

Here's a 21-day exercise plan designed specifically for women over 70 following a ketogenic lifestyle. These exercises are beginner-friendly and can be done at your own pace. Remember to consult with your healthcare provider before starting any new exercise routine:

Week 1: Getting Started

- ➤ **Day 1: 10-min gentle walk.** Begin with a slow-paced walk around your neighborhood or in a park. Maintain a comfortable pace.

- ➤ **Day 2: 10-min stretching routine.** Perform gentle stretching exercises for major muscle groups, holding each stretch for around 20 secs.

- ➤ **Day 3: 15-min balance exercises.** Stand on one leg for 10 secs, then switch to the other leg. Repeat this several times to improve balance.

- ➤ **Day 4: 10-min gentle walk.** Similar to Day 1, take a leisurely walk at your own pace.

- ➤ **Day 5: 10-min stretching routine.** Repeat the stretching routine from Day 2.

- ➤ **Day 6: 15-min bodyweight exercises.** Try simple bodyweight exercises like squats (slowly lower and raise your body) and wall push-ups (standing push-ups against a wall).

- ➤ **Day 7: Rest day**

Week 2: Building Stamina

- ➤ **Day 8: 15-min gentle walk.** Smildly increase your walking time from Day 4.
- ➤ **Day 9: 10-min stretching routine.** Repeat the stretching routine from Day 2.
- ➤ **Day 10: 20-min balance exercises and light resistance band exercises.** Use a resistance band for exercises like seated leg lifts and seated rows. Balance exercises include standing on one leg with your eyes closed.
- ➤ **Day 11: 15-min gentle walk.** Similar to Day 8, continue building walking endurance.
- ➤ **Day 12: 10-min stretching routine.** Repeat the stretching routine from Day 2.
- ➤ **Day 13: 20-min bodyweight exercises and light resistance band exercises.** Continue bodyweight exercises and resistance band exercises, including seated leg lifts, wall push-ups, and seated rows.
- ➤ **Day 14: Rest day**

Week 3: Progression

- ➤ **Day 15: 20-min gentle walk.** Smildly increase your walking time from Day 11.
- ➤ **Day 16: 15-min stretching routine.** Repeat the stretching routine from Day 2.
- ➤ **Day 17: 25-min balance exercises, light resistance band exercises, and gentle yoga.** Incorporate more balance exercises, resistance band exercises, and gentle yoga poses like the cat-cow stretch.
- ➤ **Day 18: 20-min gentle walk.** Similar to Day 15, continue building walking endurance.
- ➤ **Day 19: 15-min stretching routine.** Repeat the stretching routine from Day 2.
- ➤ **Day 20: 25-min bodyweight exercises, light resistance band exercises, and gentle yoga.** Continue with bodyweight exercises, resistance band exercises, and gentle yoga, including poses like the child's pose.
- ➤ **Day 21: Rest day**

Summary Of Practical Tips:

- ✓ Start each session with a warm-up and end with a cool-down.
- ✓ Listen to your body and modify exercises as needed.
- ✓ Stay hydrated throughout your workouts.
- ✓ Incorporate relaxation techniques like deep breathing after your sessions.
- ✓ Track your progress and celebrate small achievements.

Remember, the key is consistency and gradual progression. Adjust the plan to your comfort level, and enjoy the journey to improved fitness and well-being.

Chapter 6: Success Stories, Frequently Asked Questions (FAQs), Community & Support

6.1 Real-Life Transformations on the Ketogenic Diet

Within the pages of this book, I have the privilege of sharing with you a collection of remarkable success stories. These stories are a testament to the transformative potential of ketogenic diet for women over 70. While the stories featured here are just a glimpse into the thousands of success stories that exist, they hold the power to inspire and illuminate the possibilities that lie ahead. You probably know that I am Melinda Francis, a nutritionist, and the women whose journeys you will read about are not only my patients, but they are also individuals who have generously chosen to share their personal experiences. These stories offer a glimpse into the real-life impact of keto diet on the lives of women over 70, showcasing the resilience, determination, and vitality that can be achieved through this approach. As you read through these narratives, I hope you find inspiration and insights that resonate with your own journey toward improved health and well-being. Each story is a testament to the potential for positive change, and it is our sincere hope that they empower you to embrace the possibilities that the keto diet can bring to your life.

Mary's Journey to Vibrant Health. Meet Mary, a vibrant 75-year-old who decided to explore the ketogenic diet. She was struggling with weight management and low energy levels. After adopting a keto lifestyle, she gradually shed excess lbs. and felt more energetic than ever before. Mary's story demonstrates how age is not a barrier to achieving remarkable health improvements through the ketogenic diet.

Susan's Cognitive Enhancements. Susan, a 72-year-old woman, was concerned about her cognitive health. She experienced occasional memory lapses and wanted to find a way to support her brain function. With the ketogenic diet's focus on healthy fats and ketones as an energy source for the brain, Susan noticed improvements in her memory and cognitive performance. Her story emphasizes the potential neuroprotective benefits of this dietary approach.

Grace's Active Lifestyle. Grace, at the age of 70, was determined to lead an active life. She discovered that the ketogenic diet provided her with sustained energy levels, allowing her to enjoy daily walks, yoga sessions, and gardening. Her increased vitality and reduced hunger spikes have made maintaining an active lifestyle more achievable than ever.

Eleanor's Heart Health Journey. Eleanor, aged 78, had concerns about her heart health. She decided to try the ketogenic diet to lower her triglyceride levels and enhance her overall cardiovascular well-being. With the guidance of her healthcare provider (me), she successfully achieved these goals and experienced improved heart health.

Linda's Weight Management Success. Linda, at 71, had struggled with weight management for years. The ketogenic diet's appetite-regulating effects helped her control cravings and reduce overeating. By following a keto lifestyle, Linda achieved her weight loss goals while enjoying satisfying and nutritious meals.

Evelyn's Journey to Mental Clarity. Meet Evelyn, a 72-year-old woman who struggled with mental fog and lack of mental clarity. She decided to try the ketogenic diet as a potential solution. After transitioning to a low-carb, high-fat diet, Evelyn noticed a significant improvement in her cognitive abilities. She felt more focutilized and mentally sharp, allowing her to engage in activities she had once found challenging.

Patricia's Journey to Freedom from Medications. Patricia, at the age of 74, had been on various medications for years to manage her health conditions. She was motivated to explore alternative options and decided to embrace the ketogenic diet. With my guidance, she experienced positive changes in her health, reducing her reliance on medications and feeling more in control of her well-being.

Dorothy's Vibrant Golden Years. Dorothy, an 80-year-old woman, wanted to make the most of her golden years. She adopted the ketogenic diet to boost her energy levels and vitality. With the support of her family, Dorothy engaged in daily activities, including dancing and volunteering. Her story serves as an inspiration for those looking to maintain an active and fulfilling life well into their senior years.

Ruth's Resilience and Weight Loss. Ruth, aged 75, faced various health challenges, including weight management issues and fluctuating energy levels. Through her commitment to the ketogenic diet, she achieved resilience, lost excess weight, and felt more confident in her daily life. Ruth's story highlights the transformative effects of the ketogenic diet on both physical and emotional well-being.

Betty's Journey to Healthy Aging. Betty, at 70, embarked on a ketogenic journey to embrace healthy aging. She integrated keto-friendly foods rich in vital nutrients and found her way to improved bone health and overall vitality. Betty's story showcases the potential of the ketogenic diet to support the specific health needs of older women.

These real-life success stories illustrate how the ketogenic diet can be a transformative and empowering lifestyle choice for women over 70. They demonstrate that age is not a limitation when it comes to reaping the benefits of this dietary approach. Each woman's unique journey showcases the positive impact of the ketogenic diet on weight management, cognitive health, energy levels, heart health, and overall well-being.

6.2 Addressing Common Queries and Concerns

Having journeyed through the pages of this book, certainly you have already encountered some answers to these common questions. Yet, it is vital to revisit certain concepts because solid understanding is paramount. Repetition is the mother of learning, and by revisiting these fundamental aspects, we ensure that the knowledge is not merely absorbed but ingrained.

1. Is the Ketogenic Diet Safe for Women Over 70?

The ketogenic diet can be safe and beneficial for women over 70, but it's vital to approach it with awareness and care. Consult with a healthcare provider before starting any new diet, especially if you have underlying health conditions or are taking medications. It's crucial to ensure the diet aligns with your unique health needs.

2. Is Ketosis Safe for Seniors?

Ketosis is generally safe for seniors, but individual responses may vary. Ketosis is a metabolic state where your body burns fat for fuel instead of carbohydrates. It can provide a stable source of energy, but it's crucial to monitor your ketone levels accurately, especially when starting. Consult with a healthcare provider for personalized guidance.

3. How Can I Stay Hydrated on the Keto Diet?

The ketogenic diet can have a diuretic effect, increasing fluid loss through urine. Older women may be more susceptible to dehydration, so it's vital to maintain proper hydration levels. Aim for almost 8 to 10 teacups (64 to 80 oz.) of water per day, but individual needs may vary. Pay attention to your body's signals for thirst and stay well-hydrated.

4. Is the Keto Diet Sustainable in the Long Term?

The sustainability of the ketogenic diet varies among individuals. To make it more sustainable, explore different keto-friendly recipes and components to include variety to your meals. Find pleasure in keto cooking and experiment with flavors and textures. Remember that it's not just about the diet but also about enjoying the journey as part of your lifestyle.

5. How Can I Manage Appetite on the Ketogenic Diet?

The ketogenic diet can help stabilize blood sugar levels, reducing hunger spikes and improving appetite control. Consuming low-carb, high-fat foods can maintain stable blood sugar levels, preventing sudden cravings and promoting a feeling of fullness. This improved appetite control can make it easier for older women to manage food intake and adhere to dietary goals.

6. Can I Get Enough Nutrients on the Keto Diet?

A well-balanced ketogenic diet can provide vital nutrients. To ensure you receive an adequate intake of vitamins and minerals, incorporate a variety of non-starchy vegetables, lean proteins, and healthy fats into your diet. Consider taking supplements to cover any potential nutrient gaps, especially important for women over 70 who may have specific nutritional needs.

7. Can I Continue Enjoying Social Gatherings and Dining Out on Keto?

Navigating social gatherings and dining out while on the ketogenic diet can be manageable. Plan ahead by communicating your dietary preferences with hosts or restaurants. Be prepared with keto-friendly options, and focus on enjoying the social aspect rather than feeling restricted by your dietary choices.

8. What Strategies Can Help Prevent the "Keto Flu"?

The "keto flu" is a set of symptoms some people experience when transitioning into ketosis, like fatigue and nausea. To prevent or alleviate these symptoms, stay well-hydrated, replenish electrolytes, and get plenty of rest during the initial stages of ketosis.

9. What Role Does the Ketogenic Diet Play in Promoting Healthy Aging and Longevity?

The ketogenic diet may contribute to healthy aging and longevity in several ways. It can help control blood sugar levels, reduce inflammation, and support cognitive function. By promoting the use of fats as a primary energy source, the diet may aid in weight management and reduce the risk of age-related diseases.

10. Are There Specific Keto-Friendly Foods that Can Enhance Joint Health for Older Women?

Yes, certain keto-friendly foods can benefit joint health. Fatty fish like salmon, rich in omega-3 fatty acids, have anti-inflammatory properties that can reduce joint discomfort. Additionally, incorporating leafy greens and nuts can provide vitamins and minerals that support joint health.

11. Can the Ketogenic Diet Assist in Managing Age-Related Conditions Like Osteoporosis?

The ketogenic diet can be beneficial for bone health. Foods like leafy greens and dairy products, compatible with keto, provide calcium and vitamin D vital for maintaining strong bones. By reducing sugar and processed food intake, the diet may also help prevent bone loss.

12. What Are the Social and Emotional Benefits of the Ketogenic Diet for Older Women?

Beyond physical health, the ketogenic diet can have social and emotional benefits. Sharing dietary experiences with others can build a sense of community and support. The diet's impact on blood sugar stability may lead to improved mood and energy levels, positively influencing emotional well-being.

13. How Does the Ketogenic Diet Affect Weight Loss for Older Women?

The ketogenic diet can support weight loss in older women. By reducing carbohydrate intake and increasing healthy fats, it can promote fat burning and aid in shedding excess lbs..

14. What Are A few Common Challenges Seniors May Face on a Keto Diet?

Seniors may encounter challenges like adapting to a low-carb diet, managing electrolyte balance, and dealing with potential side effects like the "keto flu." It's important to be aware of these challenges and seek guidance when needed.

15. Can the Ketogenic Diet Help Manage Age-Related Health Conditions?

A few studies suggest that the ketogenic diet may have potential benefits for age-related conditions like cognitive decline and metabolic health. However, it's crucial to approach any dietary changes with care and medical advice.

16. Are There Keto-Friendly Foods That Support Bone Health in Older Women?

Specific keto-friendly foods, like leafy greens, dairy products, and fatty fish, can provide vital nutrients for bone health. Maintaining a balanced diet is vital for seniors to support their bone density.

17. How Does the Ketogenic Diet Impact Energy Levels and Vitality in Seniors?

The ketogenic diet may provide a stable source of energy by relying on fat as a primary fuel source. A few seniors report improved vitality and mental clarity on this diet, but individual responses may vary.

18. What Are the Key Benefits of the Keto Diet for Seniors?

The keto diet may offer benefits like weight loss, improved metabolic health, and enhanced mental clarity. It can be especially helpful for seniors looking to manage weight and maintain vitality.

19. Is the Keto Diet Suitable for Seniors With Medical Conditions?

The keto diet can be adapted to address specific health needs, but seniors with medical conditions should consult a healthcare professional. Modifications may be necessary to ensure safety and effectiveness.

20. What Are the Risks and Side Effects of the Keto Diet for Older Adults?

Potential side effects of the keto diet can include the "keto flu," digestive issues, and medication interactions. It's crucial for seniors to be aware of these risks and consult a healthcare provider.

21. How Can Seniors Transition to the Keto Diet Safely?

Seniors should start the keto diet gradually, monitor their health, and consult with a healthcare provider. Slowly reducing carb intake and increasing healthy fats can ease the transition.

6.3 Building a Supportive Network

For women over 70, embarking on the journey toward better health and embracing mindful eating is made significantly easier with the presence of a strong, supportive network. A supportive network is not just about individuals coming together; it's about creating an environment where women can share their experiences, challenges, and victories. Within this community, the wisdom accumulated over a lifetime becomes a valuable resource for everyone involved. The connections forged offer emotional support, motivation, and a sense of belonging that's vital for nurturing healthier habits.

Building Your Network

Building a network that is truly supportive and beneficial requires a strategic approach. Here are some key steps to consider:

- ✓ **Identify Your Contacts:** Start by creating a list of everyone you know, both personally and professionally. Your existing contacts are the foundation of your network.

- ✓ **Join Relevant Groups:** Seek out groups or organizations that align with your interests and professional goals. Participating in these groups can help you connect with like-minded individuals.

- ✓ **Online Networking:** Embrace online platforms, like LinkedIn, to expand your reach. Online networking allows you to connect with professionals from various backgrounds and locations. Facebook is one of the most popular social networks. Seniors can create a profile and connect with family, friends, and colleagues.

They can join groups related to their interests or hobbies to meet like-minded individuals. Zoom and Skype, video conferencing platforms, are excellent for face-to-face online meetings. Seniors can use these tools to stay in touch with loved ones or participate in virtual events and discussions. Many websites host forums where seniors can discuss various topics, share experiences, and seek advice. Examples include SeniorNet, AARP Community, and Reddit's "Over 60" subreddit. Don't hesitate to ask for assistance from family members or friends, especially tech-savvy individuals, to set up your online profiles and navigate these platforms.

- ✓ **Effective Communication:** Building a supportive network involves effective communication. Engage in conversations, share your experiences, and listen to others.

- ✓ **Reciprocity:** Remember that networking is a two-way street. Offer support and assistance to your network members, and they are likely to reciprocate.

- ✓ **Consistency:** Consistency is key to network building. Dedicate time each week to networking activities, whether it's emailing contacts, attending events, or participating in online discussions.

- ✓ **Professional Development:** Invest in your professional development. Attend workshops, seminars, and conferences to meet new people and gain valuable insights.

- ✓ **Mentoring:** Consider becoming a mentor or seeking a mentor within your network. Mentorship can be a powerful way to support others and receive guidance in return.

Here are some of the benefits of community participation and engagement:

- ✓ **Sense of Belonging:** Community involvement fosters a sense of belonging. It allows individuals to feel connected to others, reducing feelings of isolation and loneliness .

- ✓ **Psychosocial Health:** Engaging in community activities can enrich and change lives, leading to improved psychosocial health. This can include positive effects on mental well-being and emotional health.

- ✓ **Emotional Well-Being:** Building relationships with others within a community can be of central importance to individual emotional health and overall well-being. These connections contribute to a positive outlook on life.

- ✓ **Social Support:** Communities provide a support system where individuals can both give and receive social support. This support network can reduce stress, promote feelings of independence, and contribute to older adults' identities.

- ✓ **Health Benefits:** Engagement in community activities and senior centers can lead to improved health and overall well-being among older adults. Participating in community-based social innovations can empower individuals to care for themselves, improving self-efficacy.

Chapter 7: Keto Recipes For Breakfast

1.Creamy Avocado and Smoked Salmon Toast

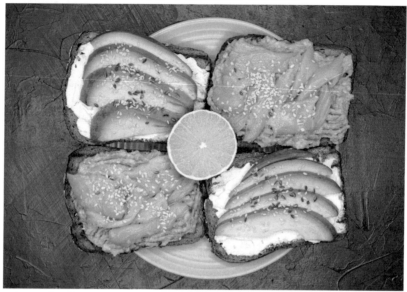

(Setup Time: 5 mins | Cooked in: 2 mins | How Many People: 2)

Recipe Components:

- 1 ripe avocado
- 2 slices of your choice of bread (e.g., whole grain, sourdough)
- 100g (3.5 oz) smoked salmon
- 2 tbsps cream cheese
- 1 lemon
- Salt and pepper as required
- Fresh dill for garnish (optional)

Preparation Steps:

- ✓ Toast the bread slices till they are golden brown to your liking.
- ✓ While the bread is toasting, cut the ripe avocado in half, take out the pit, and scoop out the flesh into a container.
- ✓ Squeeze the juice of half a lemon into the container with the avocado.
- ✓ Mash the avocado and lemon juice together till you achieve a creamy consistency.
- ✓ Season the avocado mixture with a tweak of salt and pepper as required.
- ✓ Once the toast is ready, spread a tbsp of cream cheese on each slice.
- ✓ Top the cream cheese with the creamy avocado mixture.
- ✓ Lay slices of smoked salmon on top of the avocado.
- ✓ Garnish with fresh dill if wanted.

Nutritional Info: Calories: 388 kcal, Protein: 4.9g, Carb: 12.7g, Fat: 33.4g.

2. Blueberry Chia Pudding

(Setup Time: 5 mins plus refrigeration time | How Many People: 2)

Recipe Components:

- 1/4 teacup chia seeds
- 1 teacup unsweetened almond milk (or any milk of your choice)
- 1/2 tsp vanilla extract
- 1 tbsp maple syrup or honey (adjust as required)
- 1/2 teacup fresh blueberries
- Fresh mint leaves for garnish (optional)

Preparation Steps:

- ✓ Inside a blending container, blend the chia seeds, almond milk, vanilla extract, and maple syrup or honey.
- ✓ Stir the mixture thoroughly, making sure the chia seeds are well distributed.
- ✓ Cover the container and put in the fridge it for almost 2 hrs or overnight to allow the chia seeds to absorb the liquid and create a pudding-like consistency.
- ✓ Before presenting, give the pudding a good stir to ensure it's smooth.
- ✓ Split the pudding into two presenting glasses.
- ✓ Top each presenting with fresh blueberries and garnish with mint leaves if wanted.

Nutritional Info: Calories: 210 kcal, Protein: 5g, Carb: 22g, Fat: 11g, Fiber: 11g, Sugar: 7g.

3. Spinach and Mushroom Breakfast Casserole

(Setup Time: 15 mins | Cooked in: 45 mins | How Many People: 6-8)

Recipe Components:

- 8 big eggs
- 1 teacup milk
- 1 (10 oz) package frozen severed spinach, thawed and drained
- 1 teacup carved mushrooms
- 1/2 teacup cubed onion
- 1 1/2 teacups shredded cheddar cheese
- Salt and pepper as required

Preparation Steps:

- ✓ Warm up your oven to 350 deg.F (175 deg.C) and grease a 9x13-inch baking dish.
- ✓ Inside a big blending container, whisk collectively the eggs and milk.
- ✓ Include the thawed and drained spinach, carved mushrooms, cubed onion, and 1 teacup of shredded cheddar cheese to the egg mixture.
- ✓ Season with salt and pepper as required, then mix everything thoroughly.
- ✓ Pour the mixture into the prepared baking dish.
- ✓ Spray the rest of the 1/2 teacup of shredded cheddar cheese on top.
- ✓ Bake in the warmed up oven for around 45 mins or till the casserole is set and the top is golden brown.

✓ Allow it to cool for a couple of mins before presenting.

✓ Cut into squares and serve your Spinach and Mushroom Breakfast Casserole.

Nutritional Info: Serving size: 1 square (assuming 8 presentings) - Calories: 175 kcal, Protein: 12g, Carb: 6g, Fat: 11g.

4. Cauliflower Hash Browns

(Setup Time: 15 mins | Cooked in: 20 mins | How Many People: 4)

Recipe Components:

- 1 small cauliflower head, cut into florets
- 1/4 teacup grated parmesan cheese
- 1/4 teacup shredded cheddar cheese
- 1/4 teacup almond flour
- 1 big egg
- 1/2 tsp garlic powder
- 1/2 tsp onion powder
- Salt and pepper as required
- Cooking spray or oil for frying

Preparation Steps:

✓ Begin by preheating your oven to 425 deg.F (220 deg.C) and placing a baking sheet with parchment paper.

✓ Inside a food processor, pulse the cauliflower florets till they resemble rice. Transfer the cauliflower rice to a microwave-safe container and microwave for 5 mins.

✓ Allow the microwaved cauliflower to cool and then use a clean kitchen towel to squeeze out excess moisture.

✓ Inside a blending container, blend the cauliflower, parmesan cheese, cheddar cheese, almond flour, egg, garlic powder, onion powder, salt, and pepper. Mix till all components are thoroughly mixed.

✓ Split the mixture into 4 equal portions and shape them into oval-shaped patties.

✓ Heat a griddle at med-high temp. and mildly grease with cooking spray or oil.

✓ Cook the cauliflower hash browns for around 4-5 mins on all sides, or till they are golden brown and crispy.

✓ Transfer them to the prepared baking sheet and finish baking in the oven for an extra 10 mins to ensure they are fully cooked.

✓ Serve your Cauliflower Hash Browns hot and enjoy.

Nutritional Info: Calories: 127 kcal, Protein: 7g, Carb: 7g, Fat: 9g.

5. Coconut Almond Keto Pancakes

(Setup Time: 10 mins | Cooked in: 10 mins | How Many People: 2)

Recipe Components:

- 1/2 teacup almond flour
- 2 tbsps coconut flour

- 1/2 tsp baking powder
- 2 big eggs
- 1/4 teacup unsweetened almond milk
- 2 tbsps coconut oil, dissolved
- 1/2 tsp vanilla extract
- 1-2 tbsps erythritol or your preferred keto-friendly sweetener (adjust as required)
- Pinch of salt

Preparation Steps:

- ✓ Inside a blending container, blend the almond flour, coconut flour, baking powder, and a tweak of salt.
- ✓ Inside a distinct container, whisk the eggs, almond milk, dissolved coconut oil, vanilla extract, and sweetener.
- ✓ Pour the wet components into the dry components and mix till a smooth batter forms.
- ✓ Heat a non-stick griddle or griddle at med temp. and mildly grease it with coconut oil.
- ✓ Pour 1/4 teacup of the batter onto the griddle to form each pancake. Cook for 2-3 mins on all sides, or till they are golden brown and fully cooked.
- ✓ Repeat the process till the entire batter is utilized.
- ✓ Serve your Coconut Almond Keto Pancakes with your choice of keto-friendly toppings like sugar-free syrup, berries, or whipped cream.

Nutritional Info: Calories: 330 kcal, Protein: 12g, Carb: 11g, Fiber: 6g, Net Carbs: 5g, Fat: 26g.

6. Cheddar and Chive Keto Biscuits

(Setup Time: 10 mins | Cooked in: 20 mins | How Many People: 6)

Recipe Components:

- 1 1/2 teacups almond flour
- 1/4 teacup coconut flour
- 1 1/2 tsps baking powder
- 1/2 tsp garlic powder
- 1/4 tsp salt
- 1/4 teacup chives, finely severed
- 1 1/2 teacups shredded sharp cheddar cheese
- 1/2 teacup unsalted butter, dissolved
- 3 big eggs

Preparation Steps:

- ✓ Warm up your oven to 350 deg.F (175 deg.C) and line a baking sheet with parchment paper.
- ✓ Inside a blending container, blend the almond flour, coconut flour, baking powder, garlic powder, and salt.
- ✓ Stir in the finely severed chives and shredded cheddar cheese.
- ✓ Inside a distinct container, whisk the dissolved butter and eggs together.
- ✓ Pour the wet mixture into the dry components and stir till you have a dense dough.
- ✓ Use your hands to form 6 equal-sized biscuit rounds and place them on the prepared baking sheet.

- ✓ Bake in the warmed up oven for around 20 mins or till the biscuits are golden brown and firm to the touch.
- ✓ Allow the biscuits to cool for a couple of mins before presenting.

Nutritional Info: Calories: 415 kcal, Protein: 13g, Carb: 9g, Fiber: 4g, Net Carbs: 5g, Fat: 37g.

7. Turmeric Scrambled Eggs

(Setup Time: 5 mins | Cooked in: 5 mins | How Many People: 2)

Recipe Components:

- 4 big eggs
- 1/2 tsp ground turmeric
- 1/4 tsp ground cumin
- 1/4 tsp ground coriander
- Salt and pepper as required
- 2 tbsps butter or ghee
- Fresh cilantro for garnish (optional)

Preparation Steps:

- ✓ Inside a container, whisk the eggs till well beaten.
- ✓ Include the ground turmeric, ground cumin, ground coriander, salt, and pepper to the beaten eggs. Whisk everything together till the spices are well incorporated.
- ✓ Heat the butter or ghee in a non-stick griddle at med temp.
- ✓ Pour the spiced egg mixture into the griddle.
- ✓ Stir continuously with a spatula for around 3-4 mins till the eggs are fully cooked and mildly creamy.
- ✓ Once cooked to your anticipated uniformity, take out from heat.
- ✓ Garnish with fresh cilantro if wanted.

Nutritional Info: Calories: 236 kcal, Protein: 12g, Carb: 1g, Fat: 20g.

8. Keto Strawberry Smoothie Bowl

(Setup Time: 5 mins | How Many People: 1)

Recipe Components:

- 1 teacup frozen strawberries
- 1/2 teacup unsweetened almond milk
- 1/2 tsp erythritol (or your preferred keto-friendly sweetener)
- 1/4 teacup Greek yogurt
- 1 tbsp chia seeds
- 1/2 tsp vanilla extract
- Toppings: Sliced strawberries, chia seeds, unsweetened coconut flakes, and carved almonds (optional)

Preparation Steps:

- ✓ Inside a blender, blend the frozen strawberries, unsweetened almond milk, Greek yogurt, chia seeds, vanilla extract, and erythritol.

- ✓ Blend till the mixture is smooth and creamy.
- ✓ Pour the smoothie into a container.
- ✓ Top with carved strawberries, chia seeds, unsweetened coconut flakes, and carved almonds if wanted.

Nutritional Info: Calories: 240 kcal, Protein: 8g, Carb: 20g (Net Carbs: 8g), Fiber: 12g, Fat: 14g

---

9. Bacon-Wrapped Asparagus

(Setup Time: 10 mins | Cooked in: 20 mins | How Many People: 4)

Recipe Components:

- 1 bunch of asparagus spears (about 16 spears)
- 8 slices of bacon
- 1 tbsp olive oil
- Salt and pepper as required

Preparation Steps:

- ✓ Warm up your oven to 400 deg.F (200 deg.C).
- ✓ Wash and trim the woody ends of the asparagus spears.
- ✓ Split the asparagus into bundles of 4 spears each.
- ✓ Wrap each bundle with 2 slices of bacon, securing the ends with toothpicks.
- ✓ Put the bacon-wrapped asparagus bundles on a baking sheet, spray with olive oil, and season with salt and pepper.
- ✓ Roast in the warmed up oven for around 20 mins or till the bacon is crispy, and the asparagus is soft.
- ✓ Take out the toothpicks before presenting.

Nutritional Info: Calories: 160 kcal, Protein: 5g, Carb: 4g, Fiber: 2g, Fat: 14g

---

10. Almond Flour Waffles

(Setup Time: 10 mins | Cooked in: 15 mins | How Many People: 4)

Recipe Components:

- 1 1/2 teacups almond flour
- 2 tbsps erythritol (or your preferred low-carb sweetener)
- 1/2 tsp baking powder
- 1/4 tsp salt
- 3 big eggs
- 1/2 teacup unsweetened almond milk
- 1/4 teacup dissolved butter or coconut oil
- 1 tsp vanilla extract

Preparation Steps:

- ✓ Warm up your waffle iron as per to the manufacturers guidelines.

- ✓ Inside a big container, whisk collectively the almond flour, erythritol, baking powder, and salt.
- ✓ Inside a distinct container, beat the eggs and then include the almond milk, dissolved butter (or coconut oil), and vanilla extract.
- ✓ Pour the wet components into the dry components and stir till thoroughly mixed.
- ✓ Grease the waffle iron with a little oil or cooking spray.
- ✓ Pour the waffle batter onto the warmed up waffle iron and cook till the waffles are golden brown and crisp.
- ✓ Serve the waffles with your favorite keto-friendly toppings, like sugar-free syrup or fresh berries.

Nutritional Info: Calories: 347 kcal, Protein: 11g, Carb: 8g, Fiber: 4g, Fat: 31g

11. Tomato and Basil Mini Quiches

(Setup Time: 10 mins | Cooked in: 20 mins | How Many People: 6)

Recipe Components:

- 6 big eggs
- 1/2 teacup heavy cream
- 1/2 teacup grated cheddar cheese
- 1/4 teacup fresh basil leaves, severed
- 1 teacup cherry tomatoes, halved
- Salt and pepper as required

Preparation Steps:

- ✓ Warm up your oven to 350 deg.F (175 deg.C) and grease a muffin tin or use silicone muffin teacups.
- ✓ Inside a container, whisk collectively the eggs and heavy cream till thoroughly mixed.
- ✓ Stir in the grated cheddar cheese and severed basil leaves.
- ✓ Season the mixture with salt and pepper as required.
- ✓ Pour the egg mixture evenly into the muffin teacups, filling each about halfway.
- ✓ Place one halved cherry tomato on top of each quiche.
- ✓ Bake in the warmed up oven for around 20 mins or till the quiches are set and mildly golden on top.
- ✓ Take out from the oven and let them cool for a couple of mins before presenting.

Nutritional Info: Calories: 228 kcal, Protein: 11g, Carb: 2g, Fiber: 0g, Fat: 19g

12. Mediterranean Keto Omelette

(Setup Time: 5 mins | Cooked in: 10 mins | How Many People: 2)

Recipe Components:

- 4 big eggs
- 2 tbsps heavy cream
- 1/2 teacup severed spinach
- 1/4 teacup cubed tomatoes

- 1/4 teacup crumbled feta cheese
- 2 tbsps severed Kalamata olives
- 1/4 tsp dried oregano
- Salt and pepper as required

Preparation Steps:

✓ Inside a container, whisk collectively the eggs and heavy cream till thoroughly mixed.

✓ Stir in the severed spinach, cubed tomatoes, crumbled feta cheese, and severed Kalamata olives.

✓ Season the mixture with dried oregano, salt, and pepper as required.

✓ Heat a non-stick griddle at med temp. and include a bit of cooking oil or butter.

✓ Pour half of the egg mixture into the griddle and let it cook for a couple of mins till the edges set.

✓ Gently lift the edges and tilt the griddle to let the uncooked eggs flow to the edges.

✓ When the omelette is mostly set, fold it in half and cook for an extra min till fully set.

✓ Repeat the process for the second omelette.

✓ Serve hot and garnish with additional feta, olives, and fresh oregano if wanted.

Nutritional Info: Calories: 304 kcal, Protein: 16g, Carb: 5g, Fiber: 1g, Fat: 24g

13. Keto Veggie and Cheese Frittata Muffins

(Setup Time: 10 mins | Cooked in: 20 mins | How Many People: 6)

Recipe Components:

- 6 big eggs
- 1/4 teacup heavy cream
- 1/2 teacup cubed bell peppers (red, green, or yellow)
- 1/4 teacup cubed onions
- 1/4 teacup cubed mushrooms
- 1/4 teacup shredded cheddar cheese
- 1/4 tsp garlic powder
- Salt and pepper as required

Preparation Steps:

✓ Warm up your oven to 350 deg.F (175 deg.C) and grease a muffin tin with cooking spray.

✓ Inside a blending container, whisk collectively the eggs and heavy cream till thoroughly mixed.

✓ Stir in the cubed bell peppers, onions, mushrooms, and shredded cheddar cheese.

✓ Season the mixture with garlic powder, salt, and pepper as required.

✓ Pour the egg and vegetable mixture evenly into the muffin tin.

✓ Bake in the warmed up oven for around 20 mins or till the frittata muffins are set and mildly golden on top.

✓ Allow them to cool for a couple of mins before removing them from the muffin tin.

✓ Serve these keto frittata muffins warm or at room temp.

Nutritional Info: Calories: 130 kcal, Protein: 8g, Carb: 3g, Fiber: 1g, Fat: 10g

14. Cinnamon Coconut Porridge

(Setup Time: 5 mins | Cooked in: 10 mins | How Many People: 2)

Recipe Components:

- 1/2 teacup unsweetened shredded coconut
- 1 teacup unsweetened almond milk (or any preferred low-carb milk)
- 2 tbsps ground flaxseed
- 1/2 tsp ground cinnamon
- 1/4 tsp vanilla extract
- Sweetener (e.g., erythritol or stevia) as required

Preparation Steps:

- ✓ Inside a saucepan, blend the unsweetened shredded coconut and unsweetened almond milk.
- ✓ Put the saucepan at med temp. and bring the mixture to a gentle simmer. Stir occasionally.
- ✓ Once it's simmering, decrease the temp. and let it cook for around 5 mins till it densess.
- ✓ Stir in the ground flaxseed, ground cinnamon, vanilla extract, and sweetener as required.
- ✓ Cook for an extra 2-3 mins, mixing regularly till it reaches your anticipated uniformity.
- ✓ Take out from heat and let it cool for a min.
- ✓ Serve the cinnamon coconut porridge in containers, optionally topped with extra shredded coconut and a spray of cinnamon.

Nutritional Info: Calories: 200 kcal, Protein: 3g, Carb: 7g, Fiber: 4g, Fat: 17g

15. Savory Keto Crepes

(Setup Time: 10 mins | Cooked in: 15 mins | How Many People: 2)

Recipe Components:

- 1/2 teacup almond flour
- 2 big eggs
- 1/4 teacup unsweetened almond milk (or any preferred low-carb milk)
- 1 tbsp coconut flour
- 1/4 tsp salt
- 1/4 tsp garlic powder (optional)
- 1/4 tsp dried herbs of your choice (e.g., thyme, rosemary)
- Cooking oil or butter for greasing the pan

Preparation Steps:

- ✓ Inside a container, whisk collectively almond flour, coconut flour, salt, garlic powder, and dried herbs.
- ✓ Inside an extra container, beat the eggs and then stir in the unsweetened almond milk.
- ✓ Blend the wet and dry components, mixing till a smooth batter forms.
- ✓ Heat a non-stick griddle at med temp. and mildly grease it with oil or butter.

- ✓ Pour around 1/4 teacup of the batter into the griddle, swirling it around to create a thin crepe.
- ✓ Cook for 2-3 mins till the edges start to lift, then flip and cook for an extra 1-2 mins.
- ✓ Take out the crepe from the pan and repeat the process with the rest of the batter.
- ✓ Serve your savory keto crepes with your choice of fillings, like scrambled eggs, cheese, spinach, or smoked salmon.

Nutritional Info: Calories: 210 kcal, Protein: 10g, Carb: 6g, Fiber: 3g, Fat: 16g

16. Pecan Pie Keto Oatmeal

(Setup Time: 5 mins | Cooked in: 10 mins | How Many People: 2)

Recipe Components:

- 1/2 teacup almond flour
- 2 tbsps chia seeds
- 2 tbsps severed pecans
- 1 tbsp sweetener (e.g., erythritol or stevia)
- 1/2 tsp cinnamon
- A tweak of salt
- 1 teacup unsweetened almond milk
- 1/2 tsp vanilla extract
- 1 tbsp sugar-free maple syrup (optional, for topping)

Preparation Steps:

- ✓ Inside a microwave-safe container, blend almond flour, chia seeds, severed pecans, sweetener, cinnamon, and a tweak of salt.
- ✓ Stir in unsweetened almond milk and vanilla extract.
- ✓ Microwave the mixture on high for 2 mins, stopping to stir every 30 secs to prevent clumping.
- ✓ Allow the keto oatmeal to rest for a min or two to denses.
- ✓ Spray sugar-free maple syrup on top, if wanted, before presenting.

Nutritional Info: Calories: 330 kcal, Protein: 9g, Carbs: 13g, Fiber: 9g, Fat: 26g

17. Coconut Berry Parfait

(Setup Time: 10 mins | How Many People: 2)

Recipe Components:

- 1 teacup unsweetened coconut yogurt
- 1/2 teacup fresh mixed berries (e.g., strawberries, blueberries, raspberries)
- 2 tbsps unsweetened shredded coconut
- 2 tbsps severed nuts (e.g., almonds or walnuts)
- 1 tbsp sugar-free sweetener (e.g., stevia or erythritol)
- 1/2 tsp vanilla extract

Preparation Steps:

- ✓ Inside a container, blend the unsweetened coconut yogurt with the vanilla extract and sugar-free sweetener. Mix well.
- ✓ In presenting glasses or containers, start by layering a spoonful of the coconut yogurt mixture.
- ✓ Include a layer of mixed berries on top of the yogurt.
- ✓ Spray a portion of the unsweetened shredded coconut and severed nuts over the berries.
- ✓ Repeat the layers till you fill the glasses or containers.
- ✓ Finish with a final spray of the coconut yogurt and a couple of berries on top for decoration.
- ✓ Serve instantly or put in the fridge for a refreshing and healthy dessert.

Nutritional Info: Calories: 250 kcal, Protein: 5g, Carbs: 15g, Fiber: 7g, Fat: 19g

18. Keto Zucchini Bread

(Setup Time: 15 mins | Cooked in: 50-55 mins | How Many People: 12)

Recipe Components:

- 2 teacups almond flour
- 1/4 teacup coconut flour
- 1/4 teacup unsweetened cocoa powder
- 1 1/2 tsp baking powder
- 1/2 tsp baking soda
- 1/2 tsp salt
- 1 tsp ground cinnamon
- 1/2 teacup erythritol or preferred keto sweetener
- 1/4 teacup dissolved coconut oil
- 3 big eggs
- 1 tsp vanilla extract
- 1 1/2 teacups shredded zucchini (squeezed of excess moisture)
- 1/2 teacup sugar-free chocolate chips (optional)

Preparation Steps:

- ✓ Warm up your oven to 350 deg.F (175 deg.C) and grease a 9x5-inch loaf pan.
- ✓ Inside a big blending container, blend the almond flour, coconut flour, cocoa powder, baking powder, baking soda, salt, and ground cinnamon.
- ✓ Inside an extra container, whisk collectively the erythritol, dissolved coconut oil, eggs, and vanilla extract.
- ✓ Include the wet components to the dry components and stir till thoroughly mixed.
- ✓ Gently fold in the shredded zucchini and sugar-free chocolate chips if using.
- ✓ The batter should be poured into the prepped loaf pan and the top should be smoothed down.
- ✓ Bake for 50-55 mins or till a toothpick immersed into the middle comes out clean.
- ✓ Let the zucchini bread cool in the pan for 10 mins, then transfer it to a wire stand to cool entirely.
- ✓ Slice and enjoy your keto zucchini bread.

Nutritional Info: Calories: 190 kcal, Protein: 5g, Carbs: 8g, Fiber: 3g, Sugar Alcohols: 4g, Net, Carbs: 1g, Fat: 16g

---

19. Keto Cinnamon Roll Chaffles

(Setup Time: 5 mins | Cooked in: 10 mins | How Many People: 2)

Recipe Components:

- 1 big egg
- 1/2 teacup shredded mozzarella cheese
- 2 tbsps almond flour
- 1/2 tsp baking powder

- 1/2 tsp vanilla extract
- 1 tbsp erythritol or preferred keto sweetener
- 1/2 tsp ground cinnamon
- Additional butter and cinnamon for topping

For the cream cheese glaze:

- 2 tbsps cream cheese, softened
- 1 tbsp heavy cream
- 1 tbsp erythritol or preferred keto sweetener

Preparation Steps:

✓ Warm up your waffle maker.

✓ Inside a container, whisk collectively the egg, shredded mozzarella, almond flour, baking powder, vanilla extract, erythritol, and ground cinnamon.

✓ Pour half of the chaffle batter onto the warmed up waffle maker and cook for around 4-5 mins, or till it's golden and crispy.

✓ Take out the chaffle from the waffle maker and let it cool on a wire stand.

✓ Repeat with the rest of the batter to make a second chaffle.

✓ Inside a distinct container, prepare the cream cheese glaze by mixing the softened cream cheese, heavy cream, and erythritol till smooth.

✓ Disperse a layer of butter and a spray of cinnamon on one of the chaffles, then spray with the cream cheese glaze.

✓ Put the second chaffle on top to create a sandwich.

✓ Serve your keto cinnamon roll chaffle while it's warm and enjoy!

Nutritional Info: Calories: 380 kcal, Protein: 15g, Carbs: 6g, Fiber: 2g, Sugar Alcohols: 3g, Net Carbs: 1g, Fat: 32g

20. Greek Yogurt and Walnut Parfait

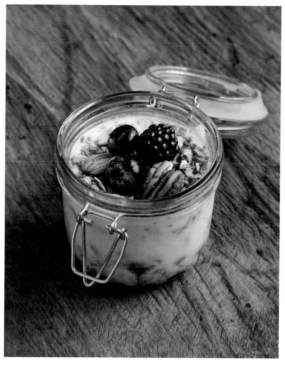

(Setup Time: 10 mins | How Many People: 2)

Recipe Components:

- 1 teacup Greek yogurt
- 1/4 teacup severed walnuts
- 1/4 teacup fresh blueberries
- 1 tbsp honey (optional)
- 1/4 tsp vanilla extract
- A tweak of cinnamon (optional)

Preparation Steps:

- ✓ Inside a container, blend Greek yogurt, vanilla extract, and honey (if wanted). Mix well.
- ✓ In presenting glasses or containers, start by layering a spoonful of the Greek yogurt mixture at the bottom.
- ✓ Include a layer of severed walnuts on top of the yogurt.
- ✓ Next, include a layer of fresh blueberries.
- ✓ Repeat the layers till the glass is filled or as desired.
- ✓ Finish with a dollop of Greek yogurt on top.
- ✓ Optionally, spray a tweak of cinnamon on the parfait for extra flavor.
- ✓ Serve instantly or put in the fridge for a cool and refreshing treat.

Nutritional Info: Calories: 280 kcal, Protein: 12g, Carbs: 16g, Fiber: 2g, Sugar: 10g, Fat: 20g

Chapter 7: Keto Recipes For Lunch

1. Keto Chicken and Vegetable Stir-Fry

(Setup Time: 10 mins | Cooked in: 15 mins | How Many People: 4)

Recipe Components:

- 1 lb. (450g) boneless, skinless chicken breasts, cut into fine strips
- 2 tbsps sesame oil
- 4 teacups (approx. 400g) mixed low-carb vegetables (e.g., broccoli, bell peppers, zucchini, snap peas)
- 3 pieces garlic, crushed
- 1/4 teacup (60ml) soy sauce (or tamari for gluten-free)
- 1 tbsp fresh ginger, crushed
- 2 tbsps rice vinegar
- 2 tbsps natural sweetener (e.g., erythritol or stevia)
- Salt and pepper as required
- Red pepper flakes (optional, for added heat)
- Fresh cilantro or green onions for garnish

Preparation Steps:

- ✓ Inside a big griddle or wok, heat 1 tbsp of sesame oil at med-high temp.
- ✓ Include the chicken strips and stir-fry till they're fully cooked and no longer pink in the center. Take out the chicken from the pan and put it away.
- ✓ Inside the same pan, include the rest of the tbsp of sesame oil. Include the crushed garlic and ginger, and sauté for around a min till fragrant.
- ✓ Include the mixed vegetables and stir-fry for 4-5 mins till they begin to soften.
- ✓ Return the cooked chicken to the pan with the vegetables.
- ✓ Inside a small container, blend collectively the soy sauce, rice vinegar, sweetener, salt, and pepper. Pour this sauce over the chicken and vegetables. If you like it spicy, include red pepper flakes at this stage.
- ✓ Continue to stir-fry for an extra 2-3 mins, allowing the sauce to cover everything evenly.
- ✓ Serve hot, garnished with fresh cilantro or green onions.

Nutritional Info: Calories: 240 kcal, Protein: 25g, Carb: 7g, Fiber: 2g, Net Carbs: 5g, Fat: 12g

2. Spinach and Feta Stuffed Chicken Breast

(Setup Time: 15 mins | Cooked in: 30 mins | How Many People: 4)

Recipe Components:

- 4 boneless, skinless chicken breasts
- 1 teacup frozen spinach, thawed and drained
- 1/2 teacup feta cheese, crumbled
- 1/4 teacup cream cheese
- 1/4 teacup grated Parmesan cheese
- 2 pieces garlic, crushed
- 1 tsp dried oregano

- Salt and pepper as required
- Olive oil for cooking

Preparation Steps:

✓ Warm up your oven to 375 deg.F (190 deg.C).

✓ Inside a blending container, blend the thawed and drained spinach, crumbled feta cheese, cream cheese, grated Parmesan cheese, crushed garlic, dried oregano, salt, and pepper. Mix well to create the stuffing mixture.

✓ Slice a pocket into the side of each chicken breast. Take cautious not to sever the whole thing with your knife.

✓ Stuff each chicken breast with the spinach and cheese mixture, evenly distributing the stuffing among them.

✓ Heat some olive oil in an ovenproof griddle at med-high temp. Put the stuffed chicken breasts in the griddle and cook for 2-3 mins on all sides till they're nicely browned.

✓ Transfer the griddle to the warmed up oven and bake for around 20-25 mins, or till the chicken is fully cooked, and the stuffing is hot and bubbly.

✓ Take out from the oven and let the chicken rest for a couple of mins before presenting.

Nutritional Info: Calories: 305, Fat: 16g, Carbohydrates: 3g, Protein: 34g

3. Greek-inspired Cucumber and Tomato Salad

(Setup Time: 15 mins | How Many People: 4)

Recipe Components:

- 4 medium-sized cucumbers, skinned and carved
- 4 big tomatoes, cubed
- 1/2 red onion, finely cut
- 1 teacup Kalamata olives, pitted and halved
- 1 teacup crumbled feta cheese
- 1/4 teacup fresh parsley, severed
- 1/4 teacup fresh mint, severed

Dressing Ingredients:

- 1/4 teacup extra-virgin olive oil
- 2 tbsps red wine vinegar
- 2 pieces garlic, crushed
- 1 tsp dried oregano
- Salt and pepper as required

Preparation Steps:

✓ Inside a big salad container, blend the carved cucumbers, cubed tomatoes, carved red onion, Kalamata olives, crumbled feta cheese, severed parsley, and severed mint.

✓ Inside a distinct small container, whisk collectively the olive oil, red wine vinegar, crushed garlic, dried oregano, salt, and pepper to make the dressing.

- ✓ Pour the dressing over the salad components in the big container.
- ✓ Shake the salad gently to ensure that all components are well covered with the dressing.
- ✓ Allow the salad to relax for around 10 mins to allow the flavors to meld together.
- ✓ Serve the Greek-inspired Cucumber and Tomato Salad as a refreshing side dish or a light main course.

Nutritional Info: Calories: 285, Fat: 23g, Carb: 15g, Protein: 6g

4. Zucchini Noodles with Pesto and Cherry Tomatoes

(Setup Time: 15 mins | Cooked in: 15 mins | How Many People: 4)

Recipe Components:

- 4 medium zucchinis
- 1 pint cherry tomatoes
- 1/2 teacup basil pesto
- 1/4 teacup grated Parmesan cheese
- Salt and pepper as required
- Red pepper flakes (optional, for heat)

Preparation Steps:

- ✓ Using a spiralizer, make zucchini noodles from the zucchinis. Put away.
- ✓ Inside a big pan, warm olive oil at med temp. Include cherry tomatoes and cook for 2-3 mins till they start to blister.
- ✓ Include the zucchini noodles to the pan, and cook for an extra 2-3 mins till they are mildly soft.
- ✓ Stir in the basil pesto and cook for an extra 2 mins, ensuring the noodles are well covered.
- ✓ Season with salt and pepper as required. If you like it spicy, include red pepper flakes.
- ✓ Serve hot, garnished with grated Parmesan cheese.

Nutritional Info: Calories: 220, Fat: 17g, Carb: 10g, Protein: 8g, Fiber: 3g

5. Keto Beef and Broccoli

(Setup Time: 10 mins | Cooked in: 20 mins | How Many People: 4)

Recipe Components:

- 1 lb. of beef sirloin, finely cut
- 4 teacups of broccoli florets
- 3 pieces of garlic, crushed
- 1/4 teacup of soy sauce (or coconut aminos for a gluten-free option)
- 2 tbsps of olive oil
- 1 tbsp of sesame oil
- 1 tbsp of erythritol or your preferred keto-friendly sweetener
- 1/2 tsp of ginger, crushed

- 1/2 tsp of xanthan gum (for densesing)
- Salt and pepper as required
- Sesame seeds and carved green onions for garnish (optional)

Preparation Steps:

- ✓ Inside a big griddle or wok, warm olive oil at med-high temp.
- ✓ Include the beef slices and cook for 2-3 mins or till browned. Take out the beef from the griddle and put it away.
- ✓ Inside the same griddle, include garlic and ginger. Sauté for around 30 secs.
- ✓ Include broccoli florets and sauté for 3-4 mins till they start to become soft.
- ✓ Inside a container, mix soy sauce, sesame oil, erythritol, and xanthan gum. Stir till thoroughly mixed.
- ✓ Return the beef to the griddle and pour the sauce over the beef and broccoli. Cook for an extra 2-3 mins till the sauce densess.
- ✓ Season with salt and pepper as required.
- ✓ Garnish with sesame seeds and carved green onions, if wanted.

Nutritional Info: Calories: 290, Fat: 20g, Carb: 7g, Fiber: 2g, Protein: 23g

6. Baked Cod with Lemon and Dill

(Setup Time: 10 mins | Cooked in: 20 mins | How Many People: 4)

Recipe Components:

- 4 cod fillets
- 2 tbsps of olive oil
- 2 pieces of garlic, crushed
- 1 lemon, finely cut
- 1/4 teacup of fresh dill, severed
- Salt and pepper as required
- Lemon wedges for presenting

Preparation Steps:

- ✓ Warm up your oven to 375 deg.F (190 deg.C). Grease a baking dish with olive oil.
- ✓ Put the cod fillets in the baking dish.
- ✓ Spray the olive oil over the fillets and season them with crushed garlic, salt, and pepper.
- ✓ Lay lemon slices on top of the cod fillets.
- ✓ Spray fresh dill over the fillets and lemon slices.
- ✓ Cover the baking dish with foil and bake for 15 mins.
- ✓ Take out the foil and bake for an extra 5 mins or till the cod is flaky and fully cooked.
- ✓ Serve with lemon wedges.

Nutritional Info: Calories: 220, Fat: 8g, Carb: 2g, Protein: 34g

7. Asparagus and Prosciutto Wraps

(Setup Time: 15 mins | Cooked in: 12 mins | How Many People: 4)

Recipe Components:

- 12 fresh asparagus spears
- 6 slices of prosciutto
- 1 tbsp olive oil
- Salt and pepper as required
- Balsamic vinegar for drizzling (optional)

Preparation Steps:

- ✓ Warm up your oven to 400 deg.F (200 deg.C).
- ✓ Trim the tough ends of the asparagus.
- ✓ Take two asparagus spears and wrap them in one slice of prosciutto, repeat for the entire asparagus.
- ✓ Put the prosciutto-wrapped asparagus on a baking sheet.
- ✓ Spray olive oil over the asparagus and season with salt and pepper.
- ✓ Roast in the warmed up oven for 10-12 mins or till the asparagus is soft and the prosciutto is crispy.
- ✓ Optionally, spray with balsamic vinegar before presenting.

Nutritional Info: Calories: 90, Fat: 6g, Carb: 2g, Protein: 7g

8. Eggplant Parmesan

(Setup Time: 30 mins | Cooked in: 40 mins | How Many People: 6)

Recipe Components:

- 2 big eggplants
- 2 teacups marinara sauce
- 2 teacups mozzarella cheese, shredded
- 1/2 teacup Parmesan cheese, grated
- 2 teacups all-purpose flour
- 3 big eggs
- 2 teacups breadcrumbs
- 2 tsps dried basil
- 2 tsps dried oregano
- Salt and pepper as required
- Olive oil for frying
- Fresh basil leaves for garnish (optional)

Preparation Steps:

- ✓ Slice the eggplants into 1/2-inch dense rounds.
- ✓ Inside a container, mix breadcrumbs with dried basil, dried oregano, salt, and pepper.
- ✓ Dredge each eggplant slice in flour, then dip into beaten eggs, and cover with the breadcrumb mixture.
- ✓ Inside a big griddle, warm olive oil at med-high temp. Fry the eggplant slices till golden brown. Put them on paper towels to drain excess oil.

- ✓ Warm up the oven to 375 deg.F (190 deg.C).
- ✓ Inside a baking dish, spread a fine layer of marinara sauce. Put a layer of fried eggplant slices, followed by mozzarella and Parmesan cheese. Repeat the layers.
- ✓ Bake in the warmed up oven for 25-30 mins or till the cheese is bubbly and golden.
- ✓ Garnish with fresh basil leaves if wanted.

Nutritional Info: Calories: 420, Fat: 19g, Carb: 45g, Protein: 18g

9. Shrimp and Cauliflower Rice Stir-Fry

(Setup Time: 10 mins | Cooked in: 15 mins | How Many People: 4)

Recipe Components:

- 1 lb. of shrimp, skinned and deveined
- 4 teacups of cauliflower rice
- 2 tbsps of oil (e.g., olive oil or sesame oil)
- Vegetables of your choice (e.g., bell peppers, broccoli, carrots)
- Sauce components (e.g., soy sauce, garlic, ginger, and optional chili flakes)
- Optional garnishes (e.g., green onions and sesame seeds)

Preparation Steps:

- ✓ Heat oil in a big griddle or wok at med-high temp.
- ✓ Include garlic and ginger, stir for around 30 secs.
- ✓ Include shrimp and stir-fry till they turn pink and opaque.
- ✓ Take out the shrimp from the griddle.
- ✓ Inside the same griddle, include more oil if needed and stir-fry your choice of vegetables till they are soft-crisp.
- ✓ Include cauliflower rice and cook for a couple of mins till it's fully heated.
- ✓ Return the shrimp to the griddle.
- ✓ Include the sauce components and stir-fry for a couple of mins till everything is thoroughly mixed and heated.
- ✓ Serve hot, garnished with green onions and sesame seeds if wanted.

Nutritional Info: Calories: 250-300 kcal, Protein: 25-30g, Carb: 10-15g, Fat: 10-15g

10. Cauliflower and Bacon Soup

(Setup Time: 15 mins | Cooked in: 35 mins | How Many People: 4)

Recipe Components:

- 1 medium-sized cauliflower head, cut into florets
- 4-6 slices of bacon, severed
- 1 onion, finely severed

- 2 pieces of garlic, crushed
- 4 teacups chicken or vegetable broth
- 1 teacup heavy cream
- Salt and pepper as required
- Chopped fresh chives for garnish (optional)

Preparation Steps:

✓ Inside a big soup pot, cook the severed bacon at med temp. till it's crispy. Take out some of the bacon bits for garnish, leaving some in the pot for flavor.

✓ Include the severed onion to the pot and cook till it's translucent.

✓ Stir in the crushed garlic and cook for an extra min.

✓ Include the cauliflower florets and sauté for a couple of mins.

✓ Pour in the chicken or vegetable broth and bring the mixture to a boil. Reduce the heat and simmer till the cauliflower is soft.

✓ Make the soup as smooth as possible by blending it with an immersion mixer. If you lack access to an immersion mixer, you may move the soup to a regular mixer in stages and puree it till it's smooth. After that, you can put it back in the pot.

✓ Stir in the heavy cream and season with salt and pepper as required.

✓ Serve hot, garnished with the reserved crispy bacon bits and severed chives if wanted.

Nutritional Info: Calories: 300-350 kcal, Protein: 8-10g, Carb: 10-15g, Fat: 20-25g

11. Avocado and Tuna Stuffed Bell Peppers

(Setup Time: 20 mins | How Many People: 2)

Recipe Components:

- 2 big bell peppers (any color)
- 1 can (5 oz) of canned tuna, drained
- 1 ripe avocado, cubed
- 1/4 teacup red onion, finely severed
- 1/4 teacup cucumber, cubed
- 2 tbsps mayonnaise
- 1 tbsp lemon juice
- Salt and pepper as required
- Fresh parsley or cilantro for garnish (optional)

Preparation Steps:

✓ Cut the tops off the bell peppers and take out the seeds and membranes. Put them away.

✓ Inside a blending container, blend the drained canned tuna, cubed avocado, severed red onion, cubed cucumber, mayonnaise, and lemon juice. Mix everything together.

✓ Season the mixture with salt and pepper as required.

✓ Stuff each bell pepper with the tuna and avocado mixture, pressing it down gently to fill the peppers.

✓ Garnish with fresh parsley or cilantro if wanted.

✓ Serve instantly, or put in the fridge till ready to serve.

Nutritional Info: Calories: 300-350 kcal, Protein: 15-20g, Carb: 10-15g, Fat: 20-25g

12. Keto Turkey and Cranberry Salad

(Setup Time: 10 mins | How Many People: 2)

Recipe Components:

- 2 teacups of cooked turkey breast, cubed
- 1/2 teacup of fresh cranberries, halved
- 1/4 teacup of severed pecans or walnuts
- 1/4 teacup of cubed celery
- 2 tbsps of mayonnaise
- 1 tbsp of Greek yogurt (optional)
- 1 tbsp of fresh lemon juice
- Salt and pepper as required
- Lettuce leaves for presenting (optional)

Preparation Steps:

✓ Inside a blending container, blend the cubed turkey breast, halved cranberries, severed nuts, and cubed celery.

✓ Inside a separate small container, mix the mayonnaise, Greek yogurt (if using), and fresh lemon juice. This will be your dressing.

✓ Pour the dressing over the turkey and cranberry mixture and shake till everything is well covered.

✓ Season with salt and pepper as required.

✓ If desired, serve the salad on a bed of lettuce leaves.

Nutritional Info: Calories: 300-350 kcal, Protein: 25-30g, Carb: 5-10g, Fat: 15-20g

13. Keto Cabbage Rolls

(Setup Time: 20 mins | Cooked in: 45-60 mins | How Many People: 4)

Recipe Components:

- 8 big cabbage leaves
- 1 lb. ground beef or ground turkey
- 1/2 teacup cauliflower rice
- 1/4 teacup cubed onion
- 1 piece garlic, crushed
- 1/4 teacup cubed tomatoes
- 1 tsp Italian seasoning
- Salt and pepper as required
- 1 teacup sugar-free tomato sauce
- 1/2 teacup beef or vegetable broth
- Shredded mozzarella cheese (optional)
- Chopped fresh parsley for garnish

Preparation Steps:

✓ Bring a big pot of water to a boil. Carefully blanch the cabbage leaves for around 2-3 mins till they are pliable. Drain and put away.

- ✓ Inside a griddle, brown the ground beef or turkey at med temp. Include cubed onion and garlic. Cook till the meat is no longer pink and the onion is translucent.
- ✓ Stir in the cauliflower rice, cubed tomatoes, Italian seasoning, salt, and pepper. Cook for an extra 5 mins.
- ✓ Warm up the oven to 350 deg.F (175 deg.C).
- ✓ Put a portion of the meat mixture in the center of each cabbage leaf. Roll them up, tucking in the sides to create rolls.
- ✓ Inside a baking dish, spread some tomato sauce on the bottom. Put the cabbage rolls in the dish.
- ✓ Pour the rest of the tomato sauce and broth over the cabbage rolls. Spray with mozzarella cheese if wanted.
- ✓ Cover with foil and bake for 45-60 mins till the cabbage is soft.
- ✓ Garnish with severed parsley before presenting.

Nutritional Info: Calories: 300-350 kcal, Protein: 20-25g, Carb: 10-15g, Fat: 10-15g

14. Thai Coconut Chicken Soup

(Setup Time: 10 mins | Cooked in: 20-25 mins | How Many People: 4)

Recipe Components:

- 1 lb. boneless, skinless chicken breasts, finely cut
- 1 can (14 oz.) coconut milk
- 4 teacups chicken broth
- 1 stalk lemongrass, cut into 2-inch pieces and smashed
- 3-4 slices galangal or ginger
- 2-3 kaffir lime leaves, torn into pieces
- 2-3 red bird's eye chilies, smashed (adjust to your preferred level of spiciness)
- 200g (about 7 oz.) white mushrooms, carved
- 1 medium tomato, cut into wedges
- 1 small onion, finely cut
- 2-3 pieces garlic, crushed
- 2-3 tbsps fish sauce (adjust as required)
- 1-2 tbsps lime juice (adjust as required)
- 1 tsp brown sugar (optional)
- Fresh cilantro leaves and carved red chilies for garnish

Preparation Steps:

- ✓ Inside a pot, bring the chicken broth to a boil. Include the lemongrass, galangal or ginger, kaffir lime leaves, and smashed red chilies. Simmer for around 10 mins to infuse the flavors.
- ✓ Include the carved chicken to the pot and simmer till it's no longer pink, around 5-7 mins. Stir in the coconut milk and let it simmer for an extra 2-3 mins.
- ✓ Include the mushrooms, tomato, onion, and garlic. Cook till the vegetables are soft, around 3-4 mins.

- ✓ Season the soup with fish sauce, lime juice, and brown sugar (if using). Adjust the seasonings to your taste.
- ✓ Take out the lemongrass, galangal or ginger, kaffir lime leaves, and smashed red chilies.
- ✓ Serve the soup hot, garnished with fresh cilantro leaves and carved red chilies.

Nutritional Info: Calories: 250-300 kcal, Protein: 25-30g, Carb: 6-8g, Fat: 15-18g

15. Spinach and Mushroom Stuffed Pork Chops

(Setup Time: 15 mins | Cooked in: 30-35 mins | How Many People: 4)

Recipe Components:

- 4 bone-in pork chops
- 1 teacup baby spinach, severed
- 1 teacup mushrooms, finely severed
- 1/2 teacup breadcrumbs
- 1/4 teacup Parmesan cheese, grated
- 2 pieces garlic, crushed
- 1/4 teacup onion, finely severed
- 1 egg
- 2 tbsps olive oil
- Salt and pepper as required
- Cooking twine (optional)

Preparation Steps:

- ✓ Warm up your oven to 375 deg.F (190 deg.C).
- ✓ Inside a griddle, heat 1 tbsp of olive oil at med temp. Include the garlic and onions and sauté till they become translucent, around 2-3 mins.
- ✓ Include the severed mushrooms and cook till they release their moisture and become soft, around 5-7 mins. Season with salt and pepper. Take out from heat and let it cool.
- ✓ Inside a blending container, blend the sautéed mushroom mixture with the severed baby spinach, breadcrumbs, grated Parmesan cheese, and the egg. Mix till all components are thoroughly mixed.
- ✓ Carefully cut a pocket into each pork chop without cutting the entire way through. Stuff each pork chop with the spinach and mushroom mixture.
- ✓ If desired, use cooking twine to secure the stuffed pork chops.
- ✓ Heat the rest of the 1 tbsp of olive oil in an oven-safe griddle at med-high temp. Brown the stuffed pork chops on both sides for around 2-3 mins on all sides.
- ✓ Transfer the griddle to the warmed up oven and bake for 20-25 mins, or till the pork reaches an internal temp. of 145 deg.F (63 deg.C) and the stuffing is golden brown.
- ✓ Let the stuffed pork chops rest for a couple of mins before presenting.

Nutritional Info: Calories: 300-350 kcal, Protein: 30-35g, Carb: 10-15g, Fat: 15-18g

16. Creamy Garlic Shrimp with Spinach

(Setup Time: 10 mins | Cooked in: 15-20 mins | How Many People: 4)

Recipe Components:

- 1 lb. big shrimp, skinned and deveined
- 2 tbsps butter
- 4 pieces garlic, crushed
- 1 teacup cherry tomatoes, halved
- 4 teacups fresh spinach
- 1 teacup heavy cream
- 1/4 teacup grated Parmesan cheese
- Salt and pepper as required
- Fresh basil leaves for garnish (optional)

Preparation Steps:

- ✓ Inside a big griddle, dissolve the butter at med-high temp. Include the crushed garlic and sauté for around 1 min, till fragrant.
- ✓ Include the shrimp to the griddle and cook for 2-3 mins on all sides or till they turn pink and opaque. Take out the cooked shrimp from the griddle and put away.
- ✓ Inside the same griddle, include the halved cherry tomatoes and cook for around 2 mins till they start to soften.
- ✓ Stir in the fresh spinach and cook till it wilts, around 2-3 mins.
- ✓ Pour in the heavy cream and grated Parmesan cheese. Stir well to blend and let it simmer for 2-3 mins, allowing the sauce to denses.
- ✓ Return the cooked shrimp to the griddle and heat through for an extra 2 mins. Season with salt and pepper as required.
- ✓ Garnish with fresh basil leaves if wanted.

Nutritional Info: Calories: 300-350 kcal, Protein: 25-30g, Carb: 6-8g, Fat: 20-25g

17. Greek Lemon Chicken Soup (Avgolemono Soup)

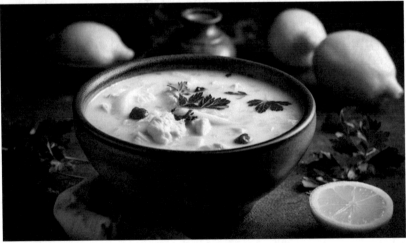

(Setup Time: 10 mins | Cooked in: 25-30 mins | How Many People: 4)

Recipe Components:

- 4 teacups chicken broth
- 2 boneless, skinless chicken breasts, cooked and shredded
- 1/2 teacup orzo pasta

- 2 big eggs
- Juice of 2 lemons
- Zest of 1 lemon
- Salt and pepper as required
- Fresh dill for garnish (optional)

Preparation Steps:

- ✓ Inside a big pot, bring the chicken broth to a boil. Include the orzo pasta and cook as per to the package guidelines till al dente.
- ✓ Once the orzo is cooked, include the shredded chicken to the pot. Let it simmer for a couple of mins.
- ✓ Inside a distinct container, whisk collectively the eggs, lemon juice, and lemon zest till thoroughly mixed.
- ✓ While continuously whisking, slowly pour a ladleful of the hot broth into the egg-lemon mixture. This tempers the eggs and prevents them from curdling.
- ✓ Slowly pour the egg-lemon mixture back into the pot with the soup, mixing regularly.
- ✓ Keep the heat low to avoid curdling.
- ✓ Continue to cook for a couple of more mins till the soup densess mildly. Season with salt and pepper as required.
- ✓ Garnish with fresh dill, if wanted.

Nutritional Info: Calories: 250-300 kcal, Protein: 20-25g, Carb: 20-25g, Fat: 5-7g

18. Keto BLT Salad

(Setup Time: 10 mins | Cooked in: 5 mins | How Many People: 4)

Recipe Components:

- 6 teacups severed romaine lettuce
- 1 teacup cherry tomatoes, halved
- 1/2 teacup cooked and crumbled bacon
- 1/4 teacup mayonnaise
- 2 tbsps sour cream
- 1 tsp Dijon mustard
- Salt and pepper as required
- Optional: grated Parmesan cheese

Preparation Steps:

- ✓ Inside a big salad containers, blend the severed romaine lettuce, halved cherry tomatoes, and crumbled bacon.
- ✓ Inside a distinct small container, whisk collectively the mayonnaise, sour cream, and Dijon mustard till thoroughly mixed.
- ✓ Season the dressing with salt and pepper as required.
- ✓ Pour the dressing over the salad and shake to cover the components evenly.
- ✓ Top the salad with grated Parmesan cheese if wanted.

Nutritional Info: Calories: 250-300 kcal, Protein: 5-7g, Carb: 5-7g, Fat: 20-25g

---

19. Spinach and Artichoke Stuffed Chicken

(Setup Time: 15 mins | Cooked in: 30-35 mins | How Many People: 4)

Recipe Components:

- 4 boneless, skinless chicken breasts
- 1 teacup frozen severed spinach, thawed and drained
- 1 teacup canned artichoke hearts, drained and severed
- 1/2 teacup cream cheese
- 1/4 teacup grated Parmesan cheese
- 2 pieces garlic, crushed
- Salt and pepper as required
- Olive oil for cooking
- Optional: additional grated Parmesan for toppinge

Preparation Steps:

- ✓ Warm up your oven to 375 deg.F (190 deg.C).
- ✓ Inside a blending container, blend the severed spinach, severed artichoke hearts, cream cheese, grated Parmesan, crushed garlic, and season with salt and pepper.
- ✓ Carefully butterfly each chicken breast by slicing horizontally through the center but not the entire way through, creating a pocket.
- ✓ Stuff each chicken breast with the spinach and artichoke mixture.
- ✓ Warm olive oil in an ovenproof griddle at med-high temp.
- ✓ Put the stuffed chicken breasts in the griddle and cook for 3-4 mins on all sides till they are nicely browned.
- ✓ Transfer the griddle to the warmed up oven and bake for 20-25 mins or till the chicken is fully cooked.
- ✓ Optional: Spray additional grated Parmesan on top of each chicken breast during the last 5 mins of baking.
- ✓ Take out from the oven, allow it to relax for a couple of mins, and serve.

Nutritional Info: Calories: 300-350 kcal, Protein: 30-35g, Carb: 5-7g, Fat: 15-20g

20. Salmon and Avocado Salad

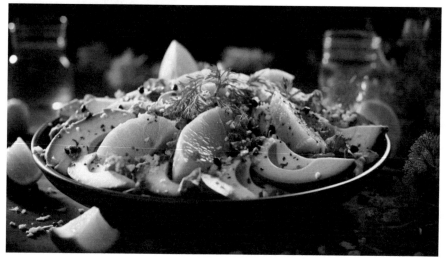

(Setup Time: 15 mins | Cooked in: 10-15 mins | How Many People: 2)

Recipe Components:

- 2 salmon fillets (about 6-8 oz. each)
- 2 tbsps olive oil
- Salt and pepper as required
- 4 teacups mixed salad greens (e.g., lettuce, spinach, arugula)
- 1 avocado, carved
- 1/2 red onion, finely cut
- 1/2 teacup cherry tomatoes, halved
- 1/4 teacup cucumber, carved
- 2 tbsps balsamic vinaigrette dressing
- Optional: lemon wedges for garnish

Preparation Steps:

- ✓ Warm up your grill or a grill pan to med-high temp.
- ✓ Brush the salmon fillets with olive oil and season with salt and pepper.
- ✓ Put the salmon fillets on the grill and cook for around 4-5 mins on all sides, or till the salmon is cooked to your desired level of doneness.
- ✓ While the salmon is cooking, prepare your salad. Inside a big container, blend the mixed salad greens, carved avocado, red onion, cherry tomatoes, and cucumber.
- ✓ Once the salmon is done, take out it from the grill and allow it to relax for a couple of mins.
- ✓ To assemble the salad, place a generous portion of the salad mixture on each plate.
- ✓ Top the salad with a grilled salmon fillet.
- ✓ Spray the balsamic vinaigrette dressing over the salad.
- ✓ Optional: Garnish with lemon wedges for added flavor.

Nutritional Info: Calories: 400-450 kcal, Protein: 30-35g, Carb: 10-15g, Fat: 25-30g

Chapter 8: Keto Recipes For Dinner

1. Creamy Spinach and Mushroom Stuffed Pork Tenderloin

(Setup Time: 15 mins | Cooked in: 40 mins | How Many People: 4)

Recipe Components:

- 1 pork tenderloin (about 1 lb.)
- 1 teacup of fresh spinach, severed
- 1 teacup of mushrooms, finely severed
- 2 pieces of garlic, crushed
- 1/2 teacup of cream cheese
- 1/4 teacup of grated Parmesan cheese
- 1 tbsp of olive oil
- Salt and pepper as required
- Kitchen twine for tying the pork

Preparation Steps:

- ✓ Warm up your oven to 375 deg.F (190 deg.C).
- ✓ Inside a griddle, warm olive oil at med temp. Include crushed garlic and sauté for around 1 min till fragrant.
- ✓ Include severed mushrooms to the griddle and cook till they release their moisture and become soft, around 5 mins. Season with salt and pepper.
- ✓ Stir in the severed spinach and cook for an extra 2 mins till it wilts. Take out the griddle from heat.
- ✓ Inside a container, blend the sautéed mushroom and spinach mixture with cream cheese and grated Parmesan. Mix well till you have a creamy filling.
- ✓ Butterfly the pork tenderloin by making a lengthwise cut down the center, without cutting the entire way through, and then open it up like a book.
- ✓ Spread the creamy spinach and mushroom mixture evenly over the inside of the pork tenderloin.
- ✓ Roll the stuffed pork tenderloin and secure it with kitchen twine at 1-inch intervals.
- ✓ Put the stuffed pork tenderloin in a baking dish and season the outside with salt and pepper.
- ✓ Roast in the warmed up oven for around 30-35 mins or till the internal temp. reaches 145 deg.F (63 deg.C).
- ✓ Take out from the oven and allow it to relax for a couple of mins before slicing.
- ✓ Slice the stuffed pork tenderloin, serve, and enjoy!

Nutritional Info: Calories: 300 kcal, Protein: 30g, Carb: 4g, Fat: 18g

2. Keto Eggplant Lasagna

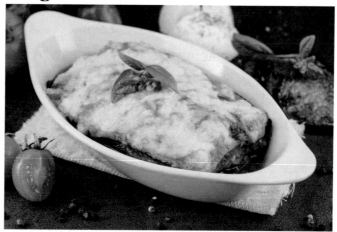

(Setup Time: 20 mins | Cooked in: 45 mins | How Many People: 6)

Recipe Components:

- 1 big eggplant, finely cut lengthwise
- 1 lb. ground beef (or ground turkey for a leaner option)
- 1/2 teacup cubed onions
- 2 pieces garlic, crushed
- 1 1/2 teacups marinara sauce (look for a low-carb version)
- 1 teacup ricotta cheese
- 1 teacup shredded mozzarella cheese
- 1/4 teacup grated Parmesan cheese
- 2 tbsps olive oil
- 1 tsp dried basil
- 1 tsp dried oregano
- Salt and pepper as required
- Fresh basil leaves for garnish (optional)

Preparation Steps:

✓ Warm up your oven to 375 deg.F (190 deg.C).

✓ Lay the carved eggplant on a baking sheet, spray with olive oil, and season with salt and pepper. Roast in the oven for around 15-20 mins or till soft. Take out and put away.

✓ Inside a griddle, warm olive oil at med temp. Include cubed onions and cook till they become translucent, around 2-3 mins. Include crushed garlic and sauté for an extra min.

✓ Include ground beef (or turkey) to the griddle and cook till browned and fully cooked. Drain any excess fat.

✓ Stir in the marinara sauce, dried basil, and dried oregano. Let it simmer for a couple of mins.

✓ Inside a distinct container, mix the ricotta cheese with a tweak of salt and pepper.

✓ Inside a baking dish, start assembling the lasagna. Begin with a layer of roasted eggplant slices, followed by a layer of the meat sauce, a layer of ricotta cheese, and a layer of mozzarella cheese. Repeat till all components are utilized.

✓ Top the lasagna with the grated Parmesan cheese.

✓ Bake in the warmed up oven for around 20-25 mins, or till the cheese is bubbly and golden.

✓ Let it cool for a couple of mins, garnish with fresh basil leaves (if wanted), slice, and serve.

Nutritional Info: Calories: 350 kcal, Protein: 25g, Carb: 9g, Fat: 24g

---

3. Dijon and Herb Crusted Salmon

(Setup Time: 10 mins | Cooked in: 15 mins | How Many People: 4)

Recipe Components:

- 4 salmon fillets
- 2 tbsps Dijon mustard
- 1/4 teacup fresh breadcrumbs (or almond flour for a low-carb option)
- 2 tbsps fresh parsley, severed
- 1 tbsp fresh dill, severed
- 2 pieces garlic, crushed
- 2 tbsps olive oil
- Salt and pepper as required
- Lemon wedges for garnish

Preparation Steps:

✓ Warm up your oven to 400 deg.F (200 deg.C).

✓ Inside a small container, blend the Dijon mustard, fresh breadcrumbs (or almond flour), fresh parsley, fresh dill, crushed garlic, olive oil, salt, and pepper. Mix well to form a crumbly mixture.

✓ Put the salmon fillets on a baking sheet lined with parchment paper.

✓ Spread the Dijon and herb mixture evenly over the top of each salmon fillet, pressing it down gently to adhere.

✓ Bake in the warmed up oven for around 12-15 mins or till the salmon flakes simply with a fork and the crust is golden.

✓ Take out from the oven, garnish with lemon wedges, and serve hot.

Nutritional Info: Cal: 300 kcal, Protein: 25g, Carb: 5g (or lower with almond flour), Fat: 20g

---

4. Keto Beef Stroganoff

(Setup Time: 10 mins | Cooked in: 20 mins | How Many People: 4)

Recipe Components:

- 1 lb. of beef sirloin or tenderloin, finely cut
- 2 tbsps of butter
- 1 small onion, finely severed
- 2 pieces of garlic, crushed
- 8 oz. of mushrooms, carved
- 1 teacup of beef broth
- 1/2 teacup of sour cream
- 1 tbsp of Dijon mustard
- 1 tbsp of Worcestershire sauce
- Salt and pepper as required
- Fresh parsley, severed, for garnish
- Cauliflower rice or zucchini noodles for presenting

Preparation Steps:

- ✓ Inside a big griddle, dissolve the butter at med temp. Include the severed onion and garlic, and sauté till they become translucent.
- ✓ Include the finely cut beef to the griddle and cook for a couple of mins till it's browned on all sides. Take out the beef from the griddle and put it away.
- ✓ Inside the same griddle, include the carved mushrooms and cook till they release their moisture and become soft.
- ✓ Return the cooked beef to the griddle with the mushrooms.
- ✓ Stir in the beef broth, sour cream, Dijon mustard, and Worcestershire sauce. Simmer the mixture for around 5-7 mins, allowing the flavors to meld and the sauce to denses. Season with salt and pepper as required.
- ✓ Serve the Keto Beef Stroganoff over cauliflower rice or zucchini noodles.
- ✓ Garnish with severed fresh parsley before presenting.

Nutritional Info: Calories: 350 kcal, Protein: 30g, Carb: 5g, Fat: 22g

5. Lemon Garlic Shrimp and Zucchini Noodles

(Setup Time: 15 mins | Cooked in: 10 mins | How Many People: 2)

Recipe Components:

- 8 oz. of big shrimp, skinned and deveined
- 2 medium-sized zucchinis
- 2 tbsps of olive oil
- 3 pieces of garlic, crushed
- Zest of 1 lemon
- Juice of 1 lemon
- 1/4 teacup of chicken or vegetable broth
- Salt and pepper as required
- Fresh parsley, severed, for garnish
- Grated Parmesan cheese (optional)

Preparation Steps:

- ✓ Using a spiralizer, create zucchini noodles from the zucchinis. Put them away.
- ✓ Inside a big griddle, warm the olive oil at med-high temp. Include the crushed garlic and sauté for around a min till fragrant.
- ✓ Include the skinned and deveined shrimp to the griddle. Cook for 2-3 mins on all sides till they turn pink and opaque. Take out the shrimp from the griddle and put them away.
- ✓ Inside the same griddle, include the zucchini noodles. Sauté for 2-3 mins till they start to soften.
- ✓ Return the cooked shrimp to the griddle with the zucchini noodles.
- ✓ Include the lemon zest, lemon juice, and chicken or vegetable broth. Cook for an extra 2-3 mins, allowing the flavors to blend.
- ✓ Season with salt and pepper as required.
- ✓ Serve the Lemon Garlic Shrimp and Zucchini Noodles in containers, garnished with fresh parsley and grated Parmesan cheese if wanted.

Nutritional Info: Calories: 250 kcal, Protein: 20g, Carb: 8g, Fat: 15g

6. Spicy Cauliflower and Chickpea Curry

(Setup Time: 15 mins | Cooked in: 30 mins | How Many People: 4)

Recipe Components:

- 1 big cauliflower, cut into florets
- 1 can (15 oz.) of chickpeas, drained and washed
- 2 tbsps of vegetable oil
- 1 big onion, finely severed
- 2 pieces of garlic, crushed
- 1-inch piece of ginger, grated
- 1 can (14 oz.) of cubed tomatoes
- 2 tbsps of curry paste (adjust to your preferred level of spiciness)
- 1 can (14 oz.) of coconut milk
- Salt and pepper as required
- Fresh cilantro, severed, for garnish
- Cooked rice or naan bread for presenting

Preparation Steps:

- ✓ Inside a big griddle, warm the vegetable oil at med temp. Include the severed onion and cook for around 5 mins till it becomes translucent.
- ✓ Include the crushed garlic and grated ginger to the griddle. Sauté for an extra 2 mins till fragrant.
- ✓ Stir in the curry paste and cook for a min to release its flavors.
- ✓ Include the cauliflower florets and chickpeas to the griddle. Cook for 5 mins, mixing irregularly.
- ✓ Pour in the cubed tomatoes and coconut milk. Bring the mixture to a gentle simmer.
- ✓ Cover the griddle and let the curry simmer for around 15-20 mins, or till the cauliflower is soft.
- ✓ Season with salt and pepper as required.
- ✓ Serve the Spicy Cauliflower and Chickpea Curry over cooked rice or with naan bread.
- ✓ Garnish with fresh cilantro.

Nutritional Info: Calories: 350 kcal, Protein: 10g, Carb: 30g, Fat: 20g

7. Pesto and Prosciutto-Wrapped Asparagus

(Setup Time: 10 mins | Cooked in: 15 mins | How Many People: 4)

Recipe Components:

- 1 bunch of fresh asparagus spears
- 4 slices of prosciutto
- 4 tbsps of pesto sauce
- Olive oil for drizzling
- Salt and black pepper as required
- Grated Parmesan cheese (optional, for garnish)

Preparation Steps:

- ✓ Warm up your oven to 400 deg.F (200 deg.C).
- ✓ Wash and trim the tough ends of the asparagus spears.
- ✓ Lay out a slice of prosciutto on a clean surface. Spread a tbsp of pesto sauce over the prosciutto slice.
- ✓ Place several asparagus spears at the edge of the prosciutto slice and roll them up in the prosciutto.
- ✓ Repeat this process for the rest of the asparagus spears.
- ✓ Put the prosciutto-wrapped asparagus on a baking sheet.
- ✓ Spray a bit of olive oil over the asparagus bundles and season with salt and black pepper.
- ✓ Bake in the warmed up oven for around 12-15 mins or till the asparagus is soft and the prosciutto is crispy.
- ✓ Garnish with grated Parmesan cheese if wanted.

Nutritional Info: Calories: 120 kcal, Protein: 6g, Carb: 3g, Fat: 10g

8. Lemon Butter Baked Cod with Herbed Tomatoes

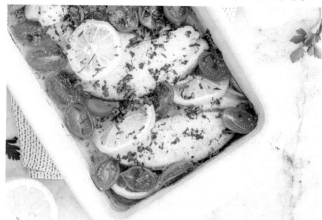

(Setup Time: 10 mins | Cooked in: 20 mins | How Many People: 4)

Recipe Components:

- 4 cod fillets
- 2 teacups cherry tomatoes, halved
- 4 tbsps unsalted butter, dissolved
- 2 pieces garlic, crushed
- Zest and juice of 1 lemon
- 2 tbsps fresh basil, severed
- 2 tbsps fresh parsley, severed
- Salt and black pepper as required
- Olive oil for drizzling

Preparation Steps:

- ✓ Warm up your oven to 375 deg.F (190 deg.C).
- ✓ Inside a baking dish, arrange the cod fillets and cherry tomato halves.
- ✓ Inside a small container, blend the dissolved butter, crushed garlic, lemon zest, and half of the lemon juice. Mix well.
- ✓ Spray the lemon butter mixture over the cod fillets and tomatoes.

- ✓ Spray the fresh basil and parsley over the top and season with salt and black pepper.
- ✓ Spray a bit of olive oil over the components.
- ✓ Bake in the warmed up oven for approximately 20 mins, or till the cod is fully cooked and the tomatoes are soft.
- ✓ Before presenting, spray the rest of the lemon juice over the dish for a fresh burst of flavor.

Nutritional Info: Calories: 240 kcal, Protein: 25g, Carb: 6g, Fat: 13g

9. Stuffed Zucchini Boats with Ground Turkey
(Setup Time: 15 mins | Cooked in: 35 mins | How Many People: 4)

Recipe Components:

- 4 medium zucchinis
- 1 lb. ground turkey
- 1 small onion, finely severed
- 2 pieces garlic, crushed
- 1 bell pepper, cubed
- 1 teacup cubed tomatoes
- 1 tsp dried oregano
- 1 tsp dried basil
- Salt and black pepper as required
- 1 teacup shredded mozzarella cheese
- Fresh parsley, for garnish

Preparation Steps:

- ✓ Warm up your oven to 375 deg.F (190 deg.C).
- ✓ Cut the zucchinis in half lengthwise and scoop out the centers to create "boats." Chop the scooped zucchini flesh and put it away.
- ✓ Inside a big griddle, heat some olive oil at med temp. Include the severed onion, garlic, and bell pepper. Sauté till they become soft.
- ✓ Include the ground turkey to the griddle and cook till it's browned and fully cooked.
- ✓ Include the cubed tomatoes, dried oregano, dried basil, salt, and black pepper to the griddle. Stir in the severed zucchini flesh. Cook for a couple of more mins till everything is thoroughly mixed.
- ✓ Fill each zucchini boat with the ground turkey mixture.
- ✓ Put the stuffed zucchini boats in a baking dish. Spray shredded mozzarella cheese over the top.
- ✓ Cover the baking dish with foil and bake for approximately 25 mins.
- ✓ Take out the foil and bake for an extra 10 mins or till the cheese is bubbly and golden.
- ✓ Garnish with fresh parsley and serve.

Nutritional Info: Calories: 280 kcal, Protein: 30g, Carb: 10g, Fat: 14g

10. Creamy Spinach and Artichoke Stuffed Chicken Breasts

(Setup Time: 20 mins | Cooked in: 25 mins | How Many People: 4)

Recipe Components:

- 4 boneless, skinless chicken breasts
- 1 teacup fresh spinach, severed
- 1/2 teacup artichoke hearts, severed
- 1/2 teacup cream cheese
- 1/4 teacup grated Parmesan cheese

- 2 pieces garlic, crushed
- 1/2 tsp dried basil
- Salt and black pepper as required
- 2 tbsps olive oil
- 1 teacup chicken broth
- Fresh parsley, for garnish

Preparation Steps:

- ✓ Warm up your oven to 375 deg.F (190 deg.C).
- ✓ Inside a blending container, blend severed spinach, severed artichoke hearts, cream cheese, grated Parmesan cheese, crushed garlic, dried basil, salt, and black pepper. Mix till thoroughly mixed.
- ✓ Carefully slice a pocket into each chicken breast. Take cautions not to sever the whole thing with your knife.
- ✓ Stuff each chicken breast with the spinach and artichoke mixture.
- ✓ Inside an ovenproof griddle, warm olive oil at med-high temp. Include the stuffed chicken breasts and cook for around 3-4 mins on all sides till they're mildly browned.
- ✓ Pour the chicken broth into the griddle.
- ✓ Transfer the griddle to the warmed up oven and bake for around 15-20 mins or till the chicken is fully cooked and no longer pink in the center.
- ✓ Garnish with fresh parsley before presenting.

Nutritional Info: Calories: 350 kcal, Protein: 30g, Carb: 6g, Fat: 20g

11. Roasted Garlic and Rosemary Lamb Chops

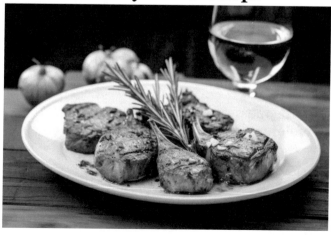

(Setup Time: 10 mins | Cooked in: 20 mins | How Many People: 4)

Recipe Components:

- 8 lamb chops
- 4 pieces of garlic, crushed
- 2 tbsps fresh rosemary, severed

- 2 tbsps olive oil
- Salt and black pepper as required
- 1 lemon, cut into wedges

Preparation Steps:

- ✓ Warm up your oven to 400 deg.F (200 deg.C).
- ✓ Inside a small container, blend the crushed garlic, severed rosemary, olive oil, salt, and black pepper.
- ✓ Rub the garlic and rosemary mixture evenly on both sides of the lamb chops.
- ✓ Heat an ovenproof griddle at med-high temp. Once hot, include the lamb chops and sear for around 2-3 mins on all sides till they're nicely browned.
- ✓ Transfer the griddle with the lamb chops to the warmed up oven.
- ✓ Roast for around 10-15 mins for medium-rare, or adjust the cooking time according to your desired level of doneness.
- ✓ Take out the lamb chops from the oven and let them rest for a couple of mins before presenting.
- ✓ Serve with lemon wedges on the side for an extra burst of flavor.

Nutritional Info: Calories: 300 kcal, Protein: 25g, Carb: 2g, Fat: 21g

12. Thai-inspired Coconut Shrimp Soup

(Setup Time: 10 mins | Cooked in: 20 mins | How Many People: 4)

Recipe Components:

- 1 lb. big shrimp, skinned and deveined
- 1 can (14 oz.) coconut milk
- 3 teacups chicken broth
- 2 stalks lemongrass, cut into 2-inch pieces and smashed
- 3-4 slices galangal or ginger
- 2-3 kaffir lime leaves
- 1-2 red chili peppers, carved (adjust to your spice preference)

- 2-3 pieces garlic, crushed
- 1 small onion, carved
- 1 teacup mushrooms, carved
- 1-2 tbsps fish sauce (adjust as required)
- 1-2 tbsps lime juice (adjust as required)
- Fresh cilantro leaves for garnish
- Salt and sugar as required

Preparation Steps:

- ✓ Inside a big pot, heat the coconut milk and chicken broth at med temp. Include lemongrass, galangal or ginger, kaffir lime leaves, and bring to a gentle simmer. Let it simmer for around 5-10 mins to infuse the flavors.

- ✓ Include the carved onion, garlic, mushrooms, and red chili peppers to the pot. Cook for around 5 mins till the vegetables are soft.
- ✓ Stir in the shrimp and let them cook for 2-3 mins till they turn pink and opaque.
- ✓ Season the soup with fish sauce, lime juice, salt, and sugar as required. Adjust the seasoning as needed.
- ✓ Take out the lemongrass, galangal or ginger, and kaffir lime leaves from the soup.
- ✓ Ladle the hot soup into presenting containers.
- ✓ Garnish with fresh cilantro leaves.

Nutritional Info: Calories: 250-300 kcal, Protein: 20-25g, Carb: 5-10g, Fat: 15-20g

13. Keto Spaghetti Squash Carbonara

(Setup Time: 15 mins | Cooked in: 45 mins | How Many People: 4)

Recipe Components:

- 1 medium-sized spaghetti squash
- 4 slices of bacon, severed
- 2 pieces garlic, crushed
- 2 big eggs
- 1/2 teacup grated Parmesan cheese
- 1/4 teacup heavy cream
- Salt and black pepper as required
- Fresh parsley for garnish (optional)

Preparation Steps:

- ✓ Warm up your oven to 375 deg.F (190 deg.C).
- ✓ Cut the spaghetti squash in half lengthwise. Scoop out the seeds and place the halves, cut side down, on a baking sheet. Roast them in the oven for around 30-40 mins or till the flesh is soft.
- ✓ While the squash is roasting, cook the severed bacon in a griddle at med temp. till it's crispy. Take out the bacon and put it away, leaving the bacon fat in the griddle.
- ✓ Inside the same griddle, include crushed garlic and sauté for a min till fragrant.
- ✓ Inside a container, whisk collectively the eggs, grated Parmesan cheese, and heavy cream.
- ✓ When the spaghetti squash is done, use a fork to scrape the flesh into "spaghetti" strands. Include the strands to the griddle with the garlic and bacon fat.
- ✓ Pour the egg and cheese mixture over the spaghetti squash, stirring quickly to blend. The heat of the squash will cook the eggs and create a creamy sauce.
- ✓ Season with salt and black pepper as required.
- ✓ Garnish with crispy bacon and fresh parsley, if wanted.

Nutritional Info: Calories: 350-400 kcal, Protein: 15-20g, Carb: 10-15g, Fat: 25-30g

14. Baked Dijon Mustard and Herb-Crusted Tilapia

(Setup Time: 10 mins | Cooked in: 15 mins | How Many People: 4)

Recipe Components:

- 4 tilapia fillets
- 2 tbsps Dijon mustard
- 1/2 teacup almond meal (or almond flour)
- 2 tbsps fresh herbs (e.g., parsley, thyme, or rosemary), finely severed
- 2 pieces garlic, crushed
- 1/4 teacup grated Parmesan cheese
- Salt and black pepper as required
- Lemon wedges for presenting

Preparation Steps:

- ✓ Warm up your oven to 375 deg.F (190 deg.C).
- ✓ Inside a shallow container, blend collectively the almond meal, fresh herbs, crushed garlic, grated Parmesan cheese, salt, and black pepper.
- ✓ Brush each tilapia fillet with a layer of Dijon mustard.
- ✓ Press each fillet into the almond meal and herb mixture, covering it evenly on both sides.
- ✓ Put the covered fillets on a baking sheet lined with parchment paper.
- ✓ Bake in the warmed up oven for around 15 mins or till the fish flakes simply with a fork and the crust is golden brown.
- ✓ Serve the Dijon Mustard and Herb-Crusted Tilapia with lemon wedges for a zesty kick.

Nutritional Info: Calories: 200-250 kcal, Protein: 25-30g, Carb: 5-10g, Fat: 10-15g

15. Cabbage and Sausage Stir-Fry

(Setup Time: 10 mins | Cooked in: 20 mins | How Many People: 4)

Recipe Components:

- 1 medium head of cabbage, finely cut
- 1 lb. sausage links, carved into rounds
- 1 onion, finely cut
- 2 pieces garlic, crushed
- 2 tbsps olive oil
- 1 tsp paprika
- Salt and black pepper as required
- Fresh parsley for garnish (optional)

Preparation Steps:

- ✓ Inside a big griddle or wok, warm the olive oil at med-high temp.
- ✓ Include the carved sausage rounds and cook till they start to brown, around 5 mins.
- ✓ Include the crushed garlic and carved onion, and sauté for an extra 3-4 mins till the onion becomes translucent.
- ✓ Spray the paprika over the sausage and vegetables, and stir well.

- ✓ Include the finely cut cabbage to the griddle and shake everything together. Cook for around 10-12 mins, or till the cabbage is soft and mildly caramelized.
- ✓ Season the stir-fry with salt and black pepper as required.
- ✓ Garnish with fresh parsley, if wanted.

Nutritional Info: Calories: 300-350 kcal, Protein: 15-20g, Carb: 10-15g, Fat: 20-25g

---

16. Keto Pork Chops with Blue Cheese Sauce

(Setup Time: 10 mins | Cooked in: 20 mins | How Many People: 4)

Recipe Components:

- 4 boneless pork chops
- Salt and black pepper as required
- 2 tbsps olive oil
- 1/2 teacup heavy cream
- 1/2 teacup blue cheese, crumbled
- 2 pieces garlic, crushed
- 1/2 teacup chicken broth
- 1 tbsp fresh parsley, severed, for garnish

Preparation Steps:

- ✓ Season the pork chops with salt and black pepper on both sides.
- ✓ Inside a big griddle, warm the olive oil at med-high temp. Include the pork chops and cook for around 4-5 mins on all sides, or till they are fully cooked and golden brown. Take out the pork chops from the griddle and put them away.
- ✓ Inside the same griddle, include the crushed garlic and sauté for around 1 min.
- ✓ Pour in the chicken broth and bring it to a simmer. Scrape up any browned bits from the bottom of the pan.
- ✓ Reduce the heat and stir in the heavy cream. Let it simmer for a couple of mins till it densess mildly.
- ✓ Include the crumbled blue cheese and stir till it dissolves into the sauce.
- ✓ Return the pork chops to the griddle and let them heat through in the sauce for a couple of mins.
- ✓ Garnish with severed fresh parsley before presenting.

Nutritional Info: Calories: 400-450 kcal, Protein: 30-35g, Carb: 2-4g, Fat: 30-35g

---

17. Keto Pesto and Mozzarella Stuffed Chicken

(Setup Time: 15 mins | Cooked in: 25 mins | How Many People: 4)

Recipe Components:

- 4 boneless, skinless chicken breasts
- Salt and black pepper as required
- 1/2 teacup keto-friendly pesto sauce
- 1 teacup mozzarella cheese, shredded
- 2 tbsps olive oil
- 1 tsp Italian seasoning (optional)

- Fresh basil leaves for garnish (optional)

Preparation Steps:

✓ Warm up your oven to 375 deg.F (190 deg.C).

✓ Place the chicken breasts on a clean surface and lay them out flat. Using a sharp knife, carefully cut a pocket into every chicken breast in a horizontal direction, taking care not to cut through to the opposite side.

✓ Season the inside of each chicken breast with salt and black pepper.

✓ Stuff each chicken breast with 2 tbsps of keto-friendly pesto sauce and 1/4 teacup of mozzarella cheese.

✓ Close the pockets by securing them with toothpicks to keep the filling in.

✓ Season the outside of each chicken breast with salt, black pepper, and Italian seasoning if wanted.

✓ Inside an ovenproof griddle, warm the olive oil at med-high temp. Include the stuffed chicken breasts and cook for around 3-4 mins on all sides or till they are golden brown.

✓ Transfer the griddle to the warmed up oven and bake for around 15-20 mins or till the chicken is fully cooked and the cheese is dissolved and bubbly.

✓ Garnish with fresh basil leaves if wanted and serve.

Nutritional Info: Calories: 350-400 kcal, Protein: 30-35g, Carb: 2-4g, Fat: 20-25g

18. Lemon Herb Shrimp and Zucchini Noodles

(Setup Time: 15 mins | Cooked in: 10 mins | How Many People: 4)

Recipe Components:

- 1 lb. big shrimp, skinned and deveined
- 4 medium zucchinis
- 2 tbsps olive oil
- 3 pieces garlic, crushed
- Zest and juice of 1 lemon
- 2 tbsps fresh basil, severed
- 2 tbsps fresh parsley, severed
- Salt and black pepper as required
- Grated Parmesan cheese for garnish (optional)

Preparation Steps:

✓ Using a spiralizer, create zucchini noodles from the zucchinis. Put them away.

✓ Inside a big griddle, warm the olive oil at med-high temp. Include the crushed garlic and sauté for around 1 min till fragrant.

✓ Include the shrimp to the griddle and cook for 2-3 mins on all sides till they turn pink and opaque. Season with salt and black pepper.

✓ Take out the cooked shrimp from the griddle and put them away.

✓ Inside the same griddle, include the zucchini noodles and cook for around 2-3 mins till they are fully heated and mildly soft.

- ✓ Return the cooked shrimp to the griddle.
- ✓ Include the lemon zest, lemon juice, fresh basil, and fresh parsley. Shake everything together to blend.
- ✓ Season with additional salt and black pepper if needed.
- ✓ Serve hot, garnished with grated Parmesan cheese if wanted.

Nutritional Info: Calories: 200-250 kcal, Protein: 20-25g, Carb: 10-12g, Fat: 8-10g

19. Beef and Broccoli Stir-Fry with Sesame Seeds

(Setup Time: 15 mins | Cooked in: 15 mins | How Many People: 4)

Recipe Components:

- 1 lb. flank steak, finely cut
- 2 teacups broccoli florets
- 2 tbsps sesame oil
- 3 pieces garlic, crushed
- 1 tbsp ginger, crushed
- 1/4 teacup low-sodium soy sauce
- 2 tbsps oyster sauce
- 1 tbsp brown sugar or a sugar substitute for a keto-friendly option
- 2 tbsps sesame seeds
- Salt and black pepper as required
- Red pepper flakes for a spicy kick (optional)
- Sliced green onions for garnish (optional)

Preparation Steps:

- ✓ Inside a container, blend the soy sauce, oyster sauce, brown sugar (or substitute), and put it away.
- ✓ Heat 1 tbsp of sesame oil in a big griddle or wok at med-high temp.
- ✓ Include the carved flank steak and stir-fry for 2-3 mins till it's browned. Take out the beef from the griddle and put it away.
- ✓ Inside the same griddle, include the rest of the sesame oil and heat it.
- ✓ Include the crushed garlic and ginger, and sauté for around 30 secs till fragrant.
- ✓ Include the broccoli florets to the griddle and stir-fry for 3-4 mins till they are soft-crisp.
- ✓ Return the cooked beef to the griddle and pour the sauce over it.
- ✓ Stir everything together and cook for an extra 2-3 mins till the sauce densess and covers the beef and broccoli.
- ✓ Season with salt, black pepper, and red pepper flakes if wanted.
- ✓ Spray sesame seeds on top and garnish with carved green onions.

✓ Serve hot over cauliflower rice or enjoy it on its own.

Nutritional Info: Calories: 300-350 kcal, Protein: 25-30g, Carb: 10-12g, Fat: 15-20g

---

20. Stuffed Avocado with Tuna and Olive Tapenade

(Setup Time: 10 mins | How Many People: 2)

Recipe Components:

- 2 ripe avocados
- 1 can (5 oz) of tuna, drained
- 2 tbsps of olive tapenade
- 1 tbsp of lemon juice
- 2 tbsps of severed fresh parsley
- Salt and black pepper as required
- Red pepper flakes for a bit of heat (optional)
- Lemon wedges for garnish (optional)

Preparation Steps:

✓ Cut the avocados in half and take out the pits. Scoop out a small portion of the flesh from each avocado half to create a hollow space for the filling.

✓ Inside a blending container, blend the drained tuna, olive tapenade, lemon juice, and severed fresh parsley. Mix well to create the filling.

✓ Season the filling with a tweak of salt and black pepper. Include red pepper flakes if you prefer a bit of heat.

✓ Stuff each avocado half with the tuna and olive tapenade filling, dividing it equally between the halves.

✓ Garnish with lemon wedges and additional severed parsley if wanted.

✓ Serve instantly as a delicious and healthy keto-friendly appetizer or light meal.

Nutritional Info: Calories: 250-300 kcal, Protein: 15-20g, Carb: 10-12g, Fat: 15-20g

Chapter 9: Keto Recipes For Dessert & Snacks

1. Coconut Almond Butter Bites

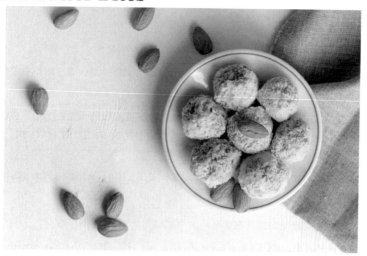

(Setup Time: 15 mins | 12 bites)

Recipe Components:

- 1/2 teacup almond butter
- 1/4 teacup unsweetened shredded coconut
- 1/4 teacup almond flour
- 2 tbsps coconut oil, dissolved
- 2 tbsps keto-friendly sweetener (e.g., erythritol or stevia)
- 1/2 tsp vanilla extract
- A tweak of salt

Preparation Steps:

- ✓ Inside a blending container, blend almond butter, unsweetened shredded coconut, almond flour, dissolved coconut oil, keto-friendly sweetener, vanilla extract, and a tweak of salt.
- ✓ Mix the entire components till they form a dough-like consistency.
- ✓ Using your hands, roll the mixture into small bite-sized balls.
- ✓ Put the bites on a parchment paper-lined tray or plate.
- ✓ Chill in the fridge for almost 30 mins to firm up.
- ✓ Once the bites have set, they are ready to enjoy.

Nutritional Info: Calories: 97, Fat: 8g, Protein: 3g, Carb: 3g, Fiber: 2g, Net Carbs: 1g

2. Pumpkin Spice Keto Cookies

(Setup Time: 15 mins | Cooked in: 12-15 mins | 12 cookies)

Recipe Components:

- 1 teacup almond flour
- 1/4 teacup canned pumpkin
- 1/4 teacup keto-friendly sweetener (e.g., erythritol or stevia)
- 1/4 teacup dissolved coconut oil
- 1 tsp pumpkin pie spice
- 1/2 tsp vanilla extract
- 1/4 tsp baking powder
- A tweak of salt

Preparation Steps:

- ✓ Warm up your oven to 350 deg.F (175 deg.C) and line a baking sheet with parchment paper.
- ✓ Inside a blending container, blend almond flour, canned pumpkin, keto-friendly sweetener, dissolved coconut oil, pumpkin pie spice, vanilla extract, baking powder, and a tweak of salt. Mix till a dough forms.
- ✓ Using your hands, form the dough into 12 small cookie shapes and put them on the prepared baking sheet.
- ✓ Gently flatten each cookie with a fork.
- ✓ Bake in the warmed up oven for 12-15 mins or till the cookies are mildly golden around the edges.
- ✓ Take out from the oven and let the cookies cool on the baking sheet for a couple of mins, then transfer them to a wire stand to cool entirely.

Nutritional Info: Calories: 90, Fat: 8g, Protein: 2g, Carb: 3g, Fiber: 1g, Net Carbs: 2g

3. Matcha Green Tea Fat Bombs

(Setup Time: 10 mins | Cooked in: 1h | 12 fat bombs)

Recipe Components:

- 1/2 teacup coconut oil
- 1/4 teacup unsweetened almond butter
- 2 tbsps matcha green tea powder
- 2 tbsps powdered Erythritol (or your preferred keto-friendly sweetener)
- 1/2 tsp vanilla extract
- A tweak of salt

Preparation Steps:

- ✓ Inside a microwave-safe container, dissolve the coconut oil and almond butter together. You can do this by microwaving in 20-second intervals till fully dissolved or using a double boiler.
- ✓ Once dissolved, stir in the matcha green tea powder, powdered Erythritol, vanilla extract, and a tweak of salt. Mix till the mixture is smooth and thoroughly mixed.
- ✓ Using a silicone mold or an ice cube tray, pour the mixture into individual mold sections. You can also use silicone molds for fun shapes.
- ✓ Put the mold in the freezer for almost 1 hr or till the fat bombs are firm.
- ✓ Once set, take out the fat bombs from the mold and store them in a sealed container in the freezer.

Nutritional Info: Calories: 90, Fat: 9g, Protein: 1g, Carb: 1g, Fiber: 1g, Net Carbs: 0g

4. Keto Peanut Butter Fudge

(Setup Time: 10 mins | Chilling: 2h | 16 pieces)

Recipe Components:

- 1 teacup natural peanut butter (unsweetened)
- 1/2 teacup coconut oil
- 1/4 teacup powdered Erythritol (or your preferred keto-friendly sweetener)
- 1/2 tsp vanilla extract
- A tweak of salt

Preparation Steps:

- ✓ Inside a microwave-safe container, dissolve the coconut oil and natural peanut butter together. You can do this by microwaving in 20-second intervals till fully dissolved or using a double boiler.
- ✓ Once dissolved, stir in the powdered Erythritol, vanilla extract, and a tweak of salt. Mix till the mixture is smooth and thoroughly mixed.
- ✓ Line a small square or rectangular dish with parchment paper, leaving some excess paper hanging over the sides for easy removal.
- ✓ Pour the peanut butter mixture into the dish and disperse it out uniformly.
- ✓ Put the dish in the fridge for around 2 hrs, or till the fudge is firm.
- ✓ Once set, use the parchment paper to lift the fudge out of the dish. Cut it into 16 equal pieces.
- ✓ Store the keto peanut butter fudge in the fridge.

Nutritional Info: Calories: 140, Fat: 12g, Protein: 4g, Carb: 3g, Fiber: 2g, Net Carbs: 1g

5. Blueberry Almond Keto Granola

(Setup Time: 10 mins | Cooked in: 25 mins | How Many People: 8)

Recipe Components:

- 1 teacup almond slices
- 1/2 teacup unsweetened shredded coconut
- 1/2 teacup chia seeds
- 1/4 teacup flaxseeds
- 1/4 teacup sunflower seeds
- 1/4 teacup pumpkin seeds
- 1/4 teacup erythritol (or your preferred keto-friendly sweetener)
- 1/4 teacup coconut oil, dissolved
- 1 tsp vanilla extract
- 1/2 teacup freeze-dried blueberries

Preparation Steps:

- ✓ Warm up your oven to 325 deg.F (160 deg.C) and line a baking sheet with parchment paper.

- ✓ Inside a big blending container, blend almond slices, unsweetened shredded coconut, chia seeds, flaxseeds, sunflower seeds, pumpkin seeds, and erythritol.
- ✓ Inside a separate microwave-safe container, dissolve the coconut oil. Stir in the vanilla extract.
- ✓ Pour the dissolved coconut oil mixture over the dry components in the big mixing container. Mix well till everything is evenly covered.
- ✓ Spread the granola mixture evenly on the prepared baking sheet.
- ✓ Bake in the warmed up oven for around 20-25 mins, or till it turns golden brown, stirring once or twice during baking for even browning.
- ✓ Take out from the oven and let the granola cool entirely on the baking sheet.
- ✓ Once the granola has cooled, break it into clusters and mix in the freeze-dried blueberries.
- ✓ Store the Blueberry Almond Keto Granola in a sealed container.

Nutritional Info: Calories: 272, Fat: 23g, Protein: 6g, Carb: 11g, Fiber: 6g, Net Carbs: 5g

6. Chocolate Mint Avocado Pudding

(Setup Time: 10 mins | How Many People: 4)

Recipe Components:

- 2 ripe avocados
- 1/4 teacup unsweetened cocoa powder
- 1/4 teacup almond milk (or any keto-friendly milk of your choice)
- 1/4 teacup keto-friendly sweetener (e.g., erythritol or stevia)
- 1/2 tsp mint extract
- A tweak of salt
- Whipped cream and fresh mint leaves for garnish (optional)

Preparation Steps:

- ✓ Cut the avocados in half, take out the pits, and scoop out the flesh into a blender or food processor.
- ✓ Include the unsweetened cocoa powder, almond milk, keto-friendly sweetener, mint extract, and a tweak of salt to the blender.
- ✓ Blend the entire components till you achieve a smooth and creamy consistency. You may need to scrape down the sides and blend again to ensure everything is well mixed.
- ✓ Taste the pudding and adjust the sweetness or mint flavor to your liking.
- ✓ Once the pudding is smooth and the taste is to your preference, transfer it to presenting dishes or teacups.
- ✓ Put in the fridge for almost 30 mins to chill and set.
- ✓ Serve chilled, optionally garnished with a dollop of whipped cream and a fresh mint leaf.

Nutritional Info: Calories: 174, Fat: 15g, Protein: 2g, Carb: 10g, Fiber: 7g, Net Carbs: 3g

7. Cinnamon Pecan Keto Brittle

(Setup Time: 10 mins | Cooked in: 20 mins | How Many People: 8)

Recipe Components:

- 1 teacup pecan halves
- 1/4 teacup unsalted butter
- 1/4 teacup keto-friendly sweetener (e.g., erythritol or stevia)
- 1 tsp ground cinnamon
- 1/4 tsp vanilla extract
- A tweak of salt

Preparation Steps:

- ✓ Warm up your oven to 325 deg.F (163 deg.C) and line a baking sheet with parchment paper.
- ✓ Inside a griddle at med temp., dissolve the unsalted butter.
- ✓ Stir in the keto-friendly sweetener, ground cinnamon, and a tweak of salt. Continue to cook and stir till the sweetener has entirely dissolved and the mixture is thoroughly mixed.
- ✓ Take out the griddle from heat and stir in the vanilla extract.
- ✓ Include the pecan halves to the griddle and cover them evenly with the cinnamon mixture.
- ✓ Spread the covered pecans onto the prepared baking sheet in a single layer.
- ✓ Bake in the warmed up oven for around 20 mins, or till the pecans are toasted and the syrup has densesed.
- ✓ Take out from the oven and let it cool entirely. As it cools, the mixture will harden and form a brittle.
- ✓ Once fully cooled and set, break the brittle into pieces.
- ✓ Store in a sealed container.

Nutritional Info: Calories: 175, Fat: 18g, Protein: 1g, Carb: 2g, Fiber: 1g, Net Carbs: 1g

8. Vanilla Chia Pudding with Berries

(Setup Time: 5 mins (plus chilling time) | How Many People: 2)

Recipe Components:

- 1/4 teacup chia seeds
- 1 teacup unsweetened almond milk (or any preferred milk)
- 1/2 tsp pure vanilla extract
- 1 tbsp keto-friendly sweetener (e.g., erythritol or stevia), or as required
- 1/2 teacup mixed berries (strawberries, blueberries, raspberries)
- Fresh mint leaves for garnish (optional)

Preparation Steps:

- ✓ Inside a blending container, blend the chia seeds, unsweetened almond milk, pure vanilla extract, and the keto-friendly sweetener. Mix well to ensure there are no clumps.

- ✓ Let the mixture sit for a couple of mins and then stir it again to prevent clumping. You can adjust the sweetness to your preference by adding more sweetener if needed.
- ✓ Cover the container and put in the fridge the chia pudding mixture for almost 2 hrs or overnight. It's ready when the chia seeds have absorbed the liquid and the mixture has densesed.
- ✓ When you're ready to serve, give the pudding a good stir. If it has densesed too much, you can include a little more almond milk to achieve your anticipated uniformity.
- ✓ Split the chia pudding into two presenting glasses.
- ✓ Top each presenting with the mixed berries and garnish with fresh mint leaves if wanted.
- ✓ Enjoy your Vanilla Chia Pudding with Berries as a delightful keto-friendly dessert or breakfast.

Nutritional Info: Calories: 150, Fat: 8g, Protein: 4g, Carb: 14g, Fiber: 10g, Net Carbs: 4g

9. Keto Cheesecake Bites

(Setup Time: 15 mins (plus chilling time) | 12 bites)

Recipe Components:

For the Crust:

- 1/2 teacup almond flour
- 2 tbsps unsweetened cocoa powder
- 2 tbsps keto-friendly sweetener (e.g., erythritol or stevia)
- 2 tbsps dissolved unsalted butter

For the Cheesecake Filling:

- 8 oz. cream cheese, softened
- 1/4 teacup keto-friendly sweetener
- 1 tsp pure vanilla extract
- 1/4 teacup heavy cream

For Topping:

- Sugar-free chocolate chips (optional)

Preparation Steps:

For the Crust:

- ✓ Inside a blending container, blend almond flour, unsweetened cocoa powder, keto-friendly sweetener, and dissolved unsalted butter. Mix till it forms a crumbly mixture.
- ✓ Line a muffin tin with cupcake liners.
- ✓ Split the crust mixture evenly among the cupcake liners, pressing it down to form the crust for each cheesecake bite.

For the Cheesecake Filling:

- ✓ Inside a distinct container, beat the softened cream cheese, keto-friendly sweetener, and pure vanilla extract till smooth and creamy.
- ✓ Include the heavy cream and mix till thoroughly mixed.
- ✓ Spoon the cheesecake filling over the crust in each cupcake liner, filling them almost to the top.

Chilling:

- ✓ If desired, spray a couple of sugar-free chocolate chips on top of each cheesecake bite.
- ✓ Put the muffin tin in the fridge and let the cheesecake bites chill for almost 2 hrs, or till they are set.
- ✓ Once set, take out them from the muffin tin and serve. Enjoy your keto cheesecake bites!

Nutritional Info: Calories: 138, Fat: 13g, Protein: 2g, Carb: 3g, Fiber: 1g, Net Carbs: 2g

---

10. Peanut Butter Chocolate Chip Keto Bars

(Setup Time: 10 mins | Cooked in: 20 mins | 12 bars)

Recipe Components:

- 1 teacup natural peanut butter (no added sugar)
- 1/4 teacup keto-friendly sweetener (e.g., erythritol or stevia)
- 1 big egg
- 1 tsp pure vanilla extract
- 1/2 teacup almond flour
- 1/4 teacup unsweetened cocoa powder
- 1/2 tsp baking powder
- 1/4 teacup sugar-free chocolate chips

Preparation Steps:

- ✓ Warm up your oven to 350 deg.F (175 deg.C) and line an 8x8-inch (20x20 cm) baking pan with parchment paper.
- ✓ Inside a blending container, blend the natural peanut butter, keto-friendly sweetener, egg, and pure vanilla extract. Mix till the entire components are well incorporated.
- ✓ Inside a distinct container, whisk collectively the almond flour, unsweetened cocoa powder, and baking powder.
- ✓ Slowly include the dry components to the peanut butter mixture and mix till a dense batter forms.
- ✓ Wrap in the sugar-free chocolate chips.
- ✓ Transfer the batter to the prepared baking pan and disperse it out uniformly.
- ✓ Bake in the warmed up oven for around 20 mins or till the edges are set, and a toothpick immersed into the middle comes out with just a couple of moist crumbs.
- ✓ Take out from the oven and allow the bars to cool in the pan for around 10 mins.
- ✓ Lift the bars out of the pan using the parchment paper and let them cool entirely on a wire stand.
- ✓ Once cool, cut into 12 bars and enjoy your Peanut Butter Chocolate Chip Keto Bars!

Nutritional Info: Calories: 170, Fat: 13g, Protein: 6g, Carb: 7g, Fiber: 3g, Net Carbs: 4g

---

11. Salted Caramel Fat Bombs

(Setup Time: 10 mins | 12 fat bombs)

Recipe Components:

- 1/2 teacup unsalted butter, softened
- 1/4 teacup coconut oil
- 1/4 teacup sugar-free caramel syrup
- 1 tsp vanilla extract
- 1/4 tsp sea salt
- 1/4 teacup almond butter
- 1/4 teacup powdered erythritol (or your preferred keto-friendly sweetener)

Preparation Steps:

- ✓ Inside a blending container, blend the softened unsalted butter, coconut oil, sugar-free caramel syrup, vanilla extract, and sea salt. Mix till the entire components are thoroughly mixed.
- ✓ Include the almond butter and powdered erythritol to the mixture. Stir till you have a smooth and creamy caramel-like mixture.
- ✓ Line a mini-muffin tin or a silicone mold with 12 cavities.
- ✓ Spoon the caramel mixture into each cavity, filling them around 2/3 full.
- ✓ Put the mold in the freezer and allow the fat bombs to set for almost 2 hrs.
- ✓ Once they are firm, take out the fat bombs from the mold and store them in a sealed container in the freezer.
- ✓ Enjoy your Salted Caramel Fat Bombs straight from the freezer as a delightful keto-friendly treat!

Nutritional Info: Calories: 118, Fat: 12g, Protein: 0.5g, Carb: 1g, Fiber: 0.5g, Net Carbs: 0.5g

---

12. Chocolate Dipped Macadamia Nut Bites

(Setup Time: 15 mins | Cooked in: 0 mins (no baking required) | 12 macadamia nut bites)

Recipe Components:

- 1 teacup roasted macadamia nuts
- 1/4 teacup sugar-free dark chocolate chips
- 1 tbsp coconut oil
- 1/2 tsp vanilla extract
- A tweak of sea salt (optional)

Preparation Steps:

- ✓ Inside a microwave-safe container, blend the sugar-free dark chocolate chips and coconut oil. Microwave in 20-second intervals, stirring between each interval, till the chocolate is fully dissolved and smooth.
- ✓ Stir in the vanilla extract and a tweak of sea salt, if wanted, into the dissolved chocolate mixture.
- ✓ Put a sheet of parchment paper on a baking sheet or tray.

- ✓ Dip each roasted macadamia nut into the chocolate mixture, ensuring it's covered evenly, and place it on the parchment paper.
- ✓ Once the entire macadamia nuts are covered, put the baking sheet in the fridge for around 20-30 mins, or till the chocolate hardens.
- ✓ Once the chocolate is set, take out the macadamia nut bites from the parchment paper, and they're ready to enjoy.
- ✓ Store any leftovers in a sealed container in the fridge.

Nutritional Info: Calories: 95, Fat: 9.5g, Protein: 1g, Carb: 2g, Fiber: 1.5g, Net Carbs: 0.5g

13. Coconut Lime Energy Bites

(Setup Time: 15 mins | Cooked in: 0 mins (no baking required) | 12 energy bites)

Recipe Components:

- 1 teacup unsweetened shredded coconut
- 1/2 teacup almond flour
- Zest and juice of 1 lime
- 2 tbsps coconut oil (dissolved)
- 2 tbsps Erythritol or your preferred keto-friendly sweetener
- 1 tsp vanilla extract
- A tweak of salt

Preparation Steps:

- ✓ Inside a blending container, blend the unsweetened shredded coconut and almond flour.
- ✓ Include the lime zest and lime juice to the dry components, followed by the dissolved coconut oil, Erythritol (or sweetener of your choice), vanilla extract, and a tweak of salt.
- ✓ Mix the components till thoroughly mixed. The mixture should be mildly sticky and simply moldable.
- ✓ Take small portions of the mixture and roll them into bite-sized balls, about 1 inch in diameter.
- ✓ Put the energy bites on a plate or tray lined with parchment paper.
- ✓ Let the energy bites set in the fridge for almost 30 mins to firm up.
- ✓ Once they've hardened, transfer them to a sealed container for storage.

Nutritional Info: Calories: 76, Fat: 7g, Protein: 1g, Carb: 3g, Fiber: 2g, Net Carbs: 1g

14. Keto Tiramisu Fat Bombs

(Setup Time: 20 mins | Cooked in: 0 mins (no baking required) | 12 fat bombs)

Recipe Components:

- 4 oz cream cheese, softened
- 4 oz mascarpone cheese
- 2 tbsps brewed and cooled espresso or strong coffee
- 2 tbsps unsweetened cocoa powder
- 2 tbsps Erythritol or your preferred keto-friendly sweetener
- 1/2 tsp vanilla extract

- 1/4 teacup crushed sugar-free ladyfingers (optional, for covering)
- Unsweetened cocoa powder for dusting (optional)

Preparation Steps:

✓ Inside a blending container, blend the softened cream cheese and mascarpone cheese. Mix till smooth and thoroughly mixed.

✓ Include the brewed and cooled espresso or coffee, unsweetened cocoa powder, Erythritol (or your sweetener of choice), and vanilla extract to the cheese mixture. Mix till all components are fully incorporated.

✓ Line a mini-muffin tin with mini-muffin liners.

✓ Scoop the mixture into the muffin liners, filling each around 3/4 full.

✓ If desired, mildly dust the tops of the fat bombs with additional unsweetened cocoa powder.

✓ Put the muffin tin in the freezer and let the fat bombs set for almost 2 hrs or till they are firm.

✓ If you choose to cover the fat bombs with crushed sugar-free ladyfingers, roll them in the crushed ladyfingers before presenting.

✓ Keep the fat bombs in the freezer till you're ready to enjoy them.

Nutritional Info: Calories: 72, Fat: 7g, Protein: 1g, Carb: 2g, Fiber: 1g, Net Carbs: 1g

---

15. Keto Cinnamon Donut Holes

(Setup Time: 15 mins | Cooked in: 15 mins | 12 donut holes)

Recipe Components:

For the Donut Holes:

- 1 teacup almond flour
- 1/4 teacup coconut flour
- 1/4 teacup granulated Erythritol or your preferred keto-friendly sweetener
- 1 tsp baking powder
- 1/4 tsp salt
- 2 big eggs
- 1/4 teacup unsweetened almond milk
- 1 tsp vanilla extract
- 2 tbsps dissolved coconut oil

For the Cinnamon Coating:

- 2 tbsps granulated Erythritol or your preferred keto-friendly sweetener
- 1 tsp ground cinnamon

Preparation Steps:

✓ Warm up your oven to 350 deg.F (175 deg.C) and line a baking sheet with parchment paper.

✓ Inside a blending container, blend the almond flour, coconut flour, granulated Erythritol, baking powder, and salt. Mix well.

- ✓ Inside a distinct container, whisk collectively the eggs, unsweetened almond milk, vanilla extract, and dissolved coconut oil.
- ✓ Pour the wet components into the dry components and stir till a dense dough forms.
- ✓ Form the dough into 12 small donut holes and place them on the prepared baking sheet.
- ✓ Bake in the warmed up oven for around 15 mins or till the donut holes are mildly golden.
- ✓ While the donut holes are baking, in a small container, blend collectively the granulated Erythritol and ground cinnamon for the covering.
- ✓ Once the donut holes are done baking, allow them to cool mildly. Then, roll each donut hole in the cinnamon covering mixture till fully covered.

Nutritional Info: Calories: 96, Fat: 7g, Protein: 3g, Carb: 6g, Fiber: 3g, Net Carbs: 3g

16. Espresso Keto Truffles

(Setup Time: 15 mins | Chilling Time: 2h | Approximately 16 truffles)

Recipe Components:

- 4 oz (115g) unsweetened chocolate, severed
- 2 tbsps unsalted butter
- 2 tbsps strong brewed espresso, cooled
- 1/4 teacup powdered erythritol (or your preferred keto-friendly sweetener)
- 1/2 tsp pure vanilla extract
- 1/8 tsp salt
- Unsweetened cocoa powder (for dusting)
- Optional toppings: crushed espresso beans, unsweetened shredded coconut, or severed nuts

Preparation Steps:

- ✓ Inside a microwave-safe container, blend the severed unsweetened chocolate and butter. Microwave in 20-second intervals, stirring in between, till the chocolate and butter are entirely dissolved and thoroughly mixed.
- ✓ Stir in the brewed espresso, powdered erythritol, vanilla extract, and salt. Mix till the sweetener is dissolved, and the mixture is smooth.
- ✓ Let the mixture cool to room temp.
- ✓ Cover the container and put in the fridge the mixture for around 1-2 hrs or till it firms up but is still pliable.
- ✓ Once the mixture is firm, use a spoon or a small scoop to portion it into approximately 16 truffles. Roll each portion into a ball using your hands.
- ✓ If desired, roll the truffles in unsweetened cocoa powder or your choice of optional toppings.
- ✓ Put the truffles on a parchment-lined tray and return them to the fridge for around 30 mins to set.
- ✓ Serve and enjoy your Espresso Keto Truffles! Store any leftovers in the fridge.

Nutritional Info: Calories: 50, Fat: 5g, Protein: 1g, Carb: 2g, Fiber: 1g, Net Carbs: 1g

17. Keto Mixed Berry Parfait

(Setup Time: 10 mins | 2 parfaits)

Recipe Components:

- 1 teacup fresh mixed berries (e.g., strawberries, blueberries, raspberries)
- 1/2 teacup full-fat Greek yogurt
- 2 tbsps almond butter
- 2 tbsps chia seeds
- 1/2 tsp vanilla extract
- 1-2 tbsps keto-friendly sweetener (adjust as required)
- 1/4 teacup severed nuts (e.g., almonds, walnuts) for topping (optional)

Preparation Steps:

✓ Inside a container, mix the full-fat Greek yogurt, almond butter, chia seeds, vanilla extract, and keto-friendly sweetener. Adjust the sweetener to your preferred level of sweetness.

✓ Wash and prepare the fresh mixed berries. If the berries are big, consider slicing them into bite-sized pieces.

✓ Take two presenting glasses or jars and begin layering your parfait. Start with a spoonful of the yogurt mixture at the bottom.

✓ Include a layer of the fresh mixed berries on top of the yogurt mixture.

✓ Repeat the layers till the glass is filled, finishing with a layer of berries on top.

✓ If desired, spray severed nuts on the very top for added texture and flavor.

✓ Chill the parfaits in the fridge for almost 30 mins to allow the chia seeds to denses the yogurt mixture.

✓ Serve the Keto Mixed Berry Parfait cold and enjoy!

Nutritional Info: Calories: 320, Fat: 20g, Protein: 12g, Carb: 18g, Fiber: 10g, Net Carbs: 8g

18. Keto Lemon Poppy Seed Muffins

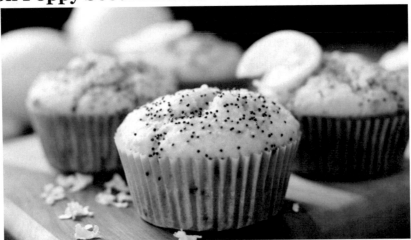

(Setup Time: 10 mins | Cooked in: 25 mins | 12 muffins)

Recipe Components:

- 2 teacups almond flour
- 1/3 teacup granulated erythritol (or any keto-friendly sweetener)
- 1 1/2 tsps baking powder
- 1 tbsp poppy seeds
- Zest of 2 lemons
- 1/4 teacup fresh lemon juice
- 3 big eggs
- 1/4 teacup unsalted butter, dissolved (or coconut oil for dairy-free)
- 1 tsp vanilla extract

Preparation Steps:

✓ Warm up your oven to 350 deg.F (175 deg.C). Line a muffin tin with paper liners or grease it.

✓ Inside a big blending container, whisk collectively the almond flour, granulated erythritol, baking powder, and poppy seeds.

✓ Inside an extra container, blend the lemon zest, lemon juice, eggs, dissolved butter, and vanilla extract.

✓ Pour the wet mixture into the dry mixture and stir till thoroughly mixed. The batter should be dense and smooth.

✓ Using a spoon or ice cream scoop, divide the batter evenly among the 12 muffin teacups.

✓ Bake in the warmed up oven for around 20-25 mins or till the muffins are golden and a toothpick immersed into the middle comes out clean.

✓ Take out the muffins from the oven and allow them to cool in the muffin tin for a couple of mins, then transfer them to a wire stand to cool entirely.

✓ Once cooled, enjoy your Keto Lemon Poppy Seed Muffins!

Nutritional Info: Calories: 180, Fat: 15g, Protein: 6g, Carb: 5g, Fiber: 2g, Net Carbs: 3g

19. Cacao Nib and Almond Butter Cups

(Setup Time: 15 mins | Cooked in: 0 mins (refrigeration time required) | 12 teacups)

Recipe Components:

- 1/2 teacup cacao nibs
- 1/4 teacup almond butter
- 2 tbsps coconut oil
- 1 tbsp powdered erythritol (or any keto-friendly sweetener)
- A tweak of salt
- 1/2 tsp vanilla extract

Preparation Steps:

✓ Inside a microwave-safe container or using a double boiler, dissolve the cacao nibs and coconut oil till smooth. This can be done by microwaving in short intervals or using a double boiler on the stove.

✓ Stir in the almond butter, powdered erythritol, salt, and vanilla extract into the dissolved cacao mixture. Mix till the entire components are thoroughly mixed.

✓ Line a mini muffin tin with 12 mini muffin liners.

- ✓ Spoon the cacao mixture evenly into each of the 12 teacups. Make sure the bottom is covered.
- ✓ Put the muffin tin in the fridge and let it set for almost 30 mins, or till the teacups are firm.
- ✓ Once set, take out the teacups from the muffin tin and enjoy your Cacao Nib and Almond Butter Cups!

Nutritional Info: Calories: 70, Fat: 6g, Protein: 2g, Carb: 3g, Fiber: 2g, Net Carbs: 1g

---

20. Keto Cinnamon Pecan Granola

(Setup Time: 10 mins | Cooked in: 25 mins | About 12 presentings)

Recipe Components:

- 1 1/2 teacups almond flour
- 1/2 teacup unsweetened shredded coconut
- 1/2 teacup severed pecans
- 1/4 teacup chia seeds
- 1/4 teacup flaxseed meal
- 1/4 teacup erythritol (or any keto-friendly sweetener)
- 1 tsp ground cinnamon
- 1/4 tsp salt
- 1/4 teacup dissolved coconut oil
- 1 big egg
- 1 tsp vanilla extract

Preparation Steps:

- ✓ Warm up your oven to 325 deg.F (160 deg.C) and line a baking sheet with parchment paper.
- ✓ Inside a big blending container, blend the almond flour, shredded coconut, severed pecans, chia seeds, flaxseed meal, erythritol, ground cinnamon, and salt.
- ✓ Inside a distinct container, whisk collectively the dissolved coconut oil, egg, and vanilla extract.
- ✓ Pour the wet mixture over the dry components and stir well till the mixture is evenly covered.
- ✓ Spread the mixture onto the prepared baking sheet and press it down to form an even layer.
- ✓ Bake in the warmed up oven for 20-25 mins or till the granola is golden brown, stirring once halfway through to ensure even cooking.
- ✓ Take out from the oven and let it cool entirely. The granola will become crisp as it cools.
- ✓ Once cooled, break the granola into clusters and store it in a sealed container.

Nutritional Info: Calories: 220, Fat: 19g, Protein: 6g, Carb: 9g, Fiber: 5g, Net Carbs: 4g

60-Day Keto Meal Plan For Women Over 70

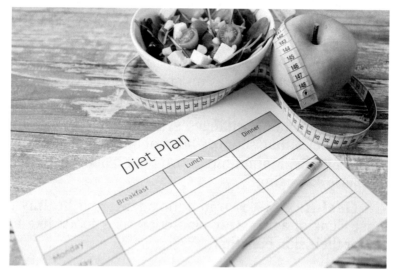

Are you ready to embark on a journey to improved health and well-being, tailored specifically for women over 70? As a seasoned nutritionist, I've meticulously designed this 60-day Keto Meal Plan to empower you on your ketogenic diet journey. This plan is not just about shedding lbs.; it's about embracing a lifestyle that enhances your vitality and overall quality of life. This meal plan isn't a one-size-fits-all approach; it's thoughtfully tailored for women over 70. We understand the unique needs and challenges you face, and this plan aims to provide a solution to meet those needs.

Why Follow Our Plan for a Ketogenic Diet?

✓ **Optimal Nutrition:** Our meal plan ensures you receive the nutrients vital for your age group, including calcium, vitamin D, and B vitamins.

✓ **Weight Maintenance:** Age can make weight management more challenging, but our plan can help you maintain a healthy weight.

✓ **Bone Health:** With a focus on calcium-rich foods, we support bone health and reduce the risk of osteoporosis.

✓ **Heart Health:** A well-structured keto diet can support cardiovascular health, an important consideration as you age.

✓ **Enhanced Cognitive Function:** A well-balanced ketogenic diet can provide a steady supply of energy to the brain, which is vital for maintaining cognitive function. Consuming foods rich in healthy fats and antioxidants may support memory, mental clarity, and overall brain health as you age.

✓ **Improved Digestive Health:** Age-related changes in digestion can lead to issues like constipation or nutrient malabsorption. Our plan comprises foods that are gentle on the digestive system, like fiber-rich vegetables and probiotic-rich options like yogurt or sauerkraut, to support gut health and regularity.

✓ **Blood Sugar Control:** A ketogenic diet can help regulate blood sugar levels. Stable blood sugar is especially important for older adults, as it can reduce the risk of diabetes and support overall well-being.

- ✓ **Reduced Inflammation:** Inflammation is linked with various age-related conditions, including arthritis and cardiovascular diseases. The anti-inflammatory properties of many foods in our meal plan, like fatty fish and leafy greens, can help reduce inflammation and promote joint and heart health.

- ✓ **Increased Energy Levels:** Many women over 70 report a decrease in energy levels. The ketogenic diet's focus on healthy fats as an energy source can provide a sustainable and steady supply of energy, which may combat feelings of fatigue.

- ✓ **Hormonal Balance:** Hormonal changes are common during the aging process. Our meal plan comprises foods that support hormonal balance, like those rich in omega-3 fatty acids and antioxidants. Maintaining hormonal balance can help manage symptoms linked with menopause and aging.

- ✓ **Enhanced Skin Health:** A diet rich in antioxidants and healthy fats can support skin health and combat signs of aging. Our plan comprises foods like avocados and berries, which are known for their skin benefits.

Day 1

Breakfast: Creamy Avocado and Smoked Salmon Toast

Lunch: Keto Chicken and Vegetable Stir-Fry

Dinner: Creamy Spinach and Mushroom Stuffed Pork Tenderloin

Snack: Coconut Almond Butter Bites

Day 2

Breakfast: Blueberry Chia Pudding

Lunch: Spinach and Feta Stuffed Chicken Breast

Dinner: Keto Eggplant Lasagna

Snack: Pumpkin Spice Keto Cookies

Day 3

Breakfast: Spinach and Mushroom Breakfast Casserole

Lunch: Greek-inspired Cucumber and Tomato Salad

Dinner: Dijon and Herb Crusted Salmon

Snack: Matcha Green Tea Fat Bombs

Day 4

Breakfast: Cauliflower Hash Browns

Lunch: Zucchini Noodles with Pesto and Cherry Tomatoes

Dinner: Keto Beef Stroganoff

Snack: Keto Peanut Butter Fudge

Day 5
Breakfast: Coconut Almond Keto Pancakes

Lunch: Keto Beef and Broccoli

Dinner: Lemon Garlic Shrimp and Zucchini Noodles

Snack: Blueberry Almond Keto Granola

Day 6
Breakfast: Cheddar and Chive Keto Biscuits

Lunch: Baked Cod with Lemon and Dill

Dinner: Spicy Cauliflower and Chickpea Curry

Snack: Chocolate Mint Avocado Pudding

Day 7
Breakfast: Turmeric Scrambled Eggs

Lunch: Asparagus and Prosciutto Wraps

Dinner: Pesto and Prosciutto-Wrapped Asparagus

Snack: Cinnamon Pecan Keto Brittle

Day 8
Breakfast: Keto Strawberry Smoothie Bowl

Lunch: Eggplant Parmesan

Dinner: Lemon Butter Baked Cod with Herbed Tomatoes

Snack: Cinnamon Pecan Keto Brittle

Day 9
Breakfast: Bacon-Wrapped Asparagus

Lunch: Shrimp and Cauliflower Rice Stir-Fry

Dinner: Stuffed Zucchini Boats with Ground Turkey

Snack: Keto Cheesecake Bites

Day 10
Breakfast: Almond Flour Waffles

Lunch: Cauliflower and Bacon Soup

Dinner: Creamy Spinach and Artichoke Stuffed Chicken Breasts

Snack: Peanut Butter Chocolate Chip Keto Bars

Day 11

Breakfast: Tomato and Basil Mini Quiches

Lunch: Avocado and Tuna Stuffed Bell Peppers

Dinner: Roasted Garlic and Rosemary Lamb Chops

Snack: Salted Caramel Fat Bombs

Day 12

Breakfast: Mediterranean Keto Omelette

Lunch: Keto Turkey and Cranberry Salad

Dinner: Thai-inspired Coconut Shrimp Soup

Snack: Chocolate Dipped Macadamia Nut Bites

Day 13

Breakfast: Keto Veggie and Cheese Frittata Muffins

Lunch: Keto Cabbage Rolls

Dinner: Keto Spaghetti Squash Carbonara

Snack: Coconut Lime Energy Bites

Day 14

Breakfast: Cinnamon Coconut Porridge

Lunch: Thai-inspired Coconut Shrimp Soup

Dinner: Baked Dijon Mustard and Herb-Crusted Tilapia

Snack: Keto Tiramisu Fat Bombs

Day 15

Breakfast: Savory Keto Crepes

Lunch: Spinach and Mushroom Stuffed Pork Chops

Dinner: Cabbage and Sausage Stir-Fry

Snack: Keto Cinnamon Donut Holes

Day 16

Breakfast: Pecan Pie Keto Oatmeal

Lunch: Creamy Garlic Shrimp with Spinach

Dinner: Keto Pork Chops with Blue Cheese Sauce

Snack: Espresso Keto Truffles

Day 17

Breakfast: Coconut Berry Parfait

Lunch: Greek Lemon Chicken Soup (Avgolemono Soup)

Dinner: Keto Pesto and Mozzarella Stuffed Chicken

Snack: Keto Mixed Berry Parfait

Day 18

Breakfast: Keto Zucchini Bread

Lunch: Keto BLT Salad

Dinner: Lemon Herb Shrimp and Zucchini Noodles

Snack: Keto Lemon Poppy Seed Muffins

Day 19

Breakfast: Keto Cinnamon Roll Chaffles

Lunch: Spinach and Artichoke Stuffed Chicken

Dinner: Beef and Broccoli Stir-Fry with Sesame Seeds

Snack: Keto Cinnamon Pecan Granola

Day 20

Breakfast: Greek Yogurt and Walnut Parfait

Lunch: Salmon and Avocado Salad

Dinner: Stuffed Avocado with Tuna and Olive Tapenade

Snack: Cacao Nib and Almond Butter Cups

Day 21

Breakfast: Keto Strawberry Smoothie Bowl

Lunch: Keto Turkey and Cranberry Salad

Dinner: Lemon Garlic Shrimp and Zucchini Noodles

Snack: Keto Cheesecake Bites

Day 22

Breakfast: Bacon-Wrapped Asparagus

Lunch: Keto Cabbage Rolls

Dinner: Spicy Cauliflower and Chickpea Curry

Snack: Peanut Butter Chocolate Chip Keto Bars

Day 23

Breakfast: Tomato and Basil Mini Quiches

Lunch: Thai Coconut Chicken Soup

Dinner: Pesto and Prosciutto-Wrapped Asparagus

Snack: Salted Caramel Fat Bombs

Day 24

Breakfast: Coconut Almond Keto Pancakes

Lunch: Spinach and Mushroom Stuffed Pork Chops

Dinner: Lemon Butter Baked Cod with Herbed Tomatoes

Snack: Chocolate Dipped Macadamia Nut Bites

Day 25

Breakfast: Blueberry Chia Pudding

Lunch: Creamy Garlic Shrimp with Spinach

Dinner: Stuffed Zucchini Boats with Ground Turkey

Snack: Coconut Lime Energy Bites

Day 26

Breakfast: Mediterranean Keto Omelette

Lunch: Greek Lemon Chicken Soup (Avgolemono Soup)

Dinner: Creamy Spinach and Artichoke Stuffed Chicken Breasts

Snack: Keto Tiramisu Fat Bombs

Day 27

Breakfast: Cinnamon Coconut Porridge

Lunch: Keto BLT Salad

Dinner: Roasted Garlic and Rosemary Lamb Chops

Snack: Keto Cinnamon Donut Holes

Day 28

Breakfast: Keto Veggie and Cheese Frittata Muffins

Lunch: Spinach and Artichoke Stuffed Chicken

Dinner: Thai-inspired Coconut Shrimp Soup

Snack: Espresso Keto Truffles

Day 29

Breakfast: Pecan Pie Keto Oatmeal

Lunch: Salmon and Avocado Salad

Dinner: Keto Spaghetti Squash Carbonara

Snack: Keto Mixed Berry Parfait

Day 30

Breakfast: Coconut Berry Parfait

Lunch: Creamy Spinach and Mushroom Stuffed Pork Tenderloin

Dinner: Baked Dijon Mustard and Herb-Crusted Tilapia

Snack: Keto Lemon Poppy Seed Muffins

Day 31

Breakfast: Blueberry Almond Keto Granola

Lunch: Cabbage and Sausage Stir-Fry

Dinner: Keto Pork Chops with Blue Cheese Sauce

Snack: Chocolate Dipped Macadamia Nut Bites

Day 32

Breakfast: Keto Cinnamon Roll Chaffles

Lunch: Thai Coconut Chicken Soup

Dinner: Stuffed Zucchini Boats with Ground Turkey

Snack: Keto Cheesecake Bites

Day 33

Breakfast: Savory Keto Crepes

Lunch: Spinach and Mushroom Stuffed Pork Chops

Dinner: Creamy Spinach and Artichoke Stuffed Chicken Breasts

Snack: Peanut Butter Chocolate Chip Keto Bars

Day 34

Breakfast: Coconut Almond Keto Pancakes

Lunch: Greek-inspired Cucumber and Tomato Salad

Dinner: Pesto and Prosciutto-Wrapped Asparagus

Snack: Salted Caramel Fat Bombs

Day 35

Breakfast: Bacon-Wrapped Asparagus

Lunch: Zucchini Noodles with Pesto and Cherry Tomatoes

Dinner: Lemon Butter Baked Cod with Herbed Tomatoes

Snack: Chocolate Dipped Macadamia Nut Bites

Day 36

Breakfast: Keto Strawberry Smoothie Bowl

Lunch: Keto Beef and Broccoli

Dinner: Stuffed Avocado with Tuna and Olive Tapenade

Snack: Keto Tiramisu Fat Bombs

Day 37

Breakfast: Mediterranean Keto Omelette

Lunch: Asparagus and Prosciutto Wraps

Dinner: Beef and Broccoli Stir-Fry with Sesame Seeds

Snack: Cacao Nib and Almond Butter Cups

Day 38

Breakfast: Keto Veggie and Cheese Frittata Muffins

Lunch: Eggplant Parmesan

Dinner: Keto Spaghetti Squash Carbonara

Snack: Keto Peanut Butter Fudge

Day 39

Breakfast: Cinnamon Coconut Porridge

Lunch: Shrimp and Cauliflower Rice Stir-Fry

Dinner: Baked Dijon Mustard and Herb-Crusted Tilapia

Snack: Coconut Almond Butter Bites

Day 40

Breakfast: Almond Flour Waffles

Lunch: Cauliflower and Bacon Soup

Dinner: Cabbage and Sausage Stir-Fry

Snack: Pumpkin Spice Keto Cookies

Day 41

Breakfast: Tomato and Basil Mini Quiches

Lunch: Avocado and Tuna Stuffed Bell Peppers

Dinner: Keto Pork Chops with Blue Cheese Sauce

Snack: Blueberry Almond Keto Granola

Day 42

Breakfast: Creamy Avocado and Smoked Salmon Toast

Lunch: Keto Turkey and Cranberry Salad

Dinner: Lemon Garlic Shrimp and Zucchini Noodles

Snack: Matcha Green Tea Fat Bombs

Day 43

Breakfast: Spinach and Mushroom Breakfast Casserole

Lunch: Keto Cabbage Rolls

Dinner: Spicy Cauliflower and Chickpea Curry

Snack: Keto Cheesecake Bites

Day 44

Breakfast: Cauliflower Hash Browns

Lunch: Thai Coconut Chicken Soup

Dinner: Pesto and Prosciutto-Wrapped Asparagus

Snack: Peanut Butter Chocolate Chip Keto Bars

Day 45

Breakfast: Cheddar and Chive Keto Biscuits

Lunch: Spinach and Artichoke Stuffed Chicken

Dinner: Lemon Herb Shrimp and Zucchini Noodles

Snack: Salted Caramel Fat Bombs

Day 46

Breakfast: Turmeric Scrambled Eggs

Lunch: Salmon and Avocado Salad

Dinner: Stuffed Avocado with Tuna and Olive Tapenade

Snack: Chocolate Dipped Macadamia Nut Bites

Day 47

Breakfast: Keto Strawberry Smoothie Bowl

Lunch: Creamy Spinach and Mushroom Stuffed Pork Tenderloin

Dinner: Keto Beef Stroganoff

Snack: Coconut Lime Energy Bites

Day 48

Breakfast: Bacon-Wrapped Asparagus

Lunch: Keto Eggplant Lasagna

Dinner: Lemon Butter Baked Cod with Herbed Tomatoes

Snack: Keto Tiramisu Fat Bombs

Day 49

Breakfast: Almond Flour Waffles

Lunch: Dijon and Herb Crusted Salmon

Dinner: Stuffed Zucchini Boats with Ground Turkey

Snack: Keto Mixed Berry Parfait

Day 50

Breakfast: Tomato and Basil Mini Quiches

Lunch: Keto Spaghetti Squash Carbonara

Dinner: Creamy Spinach and Artichoke Stuffed Chicken Breasts

Snack: Keto Lemon Poppy Seed Muffins

Day 51

Breakfast: Spinach and Mushroom Breakfast Casserole

Lunch: Baked Dijon Mustard and Herb-Crusted Tilapia

Dinner: Roasted Garlic and Rosemary Lamb Chops

Snack: Keto Cinnamon Donut Holes

Day 52

Breakfast: Pecan Pie Keto Oatmeal

Lunch: Cabbage and Sausage Stir-Fry

Dinner: Thai-inspired Coconut Shrimp Soup

Snack: Espresso Keto Truffles

Day 53

Breakfast: Coconut Berry Parfait

Lunch: Keto Pork Chops with Blue Cheese Sauce

Dinner: Keto Pesto and Mozzarella Stuffed Chicken

Snack: Keto Cinnamon Pecan Granola

Day 54

Breakfast: Keto Zucchini Bread

Lunch: Lemon Herb Shrimp and Zucchini Noodles

Dinner: Lemon Garlic Shrimp and Zucchini Noodles

Snack: Coconut Almond Butter Bites

Day 55

Breakfast: Keto Cinnamon Roll Chaffles

Lunch: Beef and Broccoli Stir-Fry with Sesame Seeds

Dinner: Stuffed Avocado with Tuna and Olive Tapenade

Snack: Pumpkin Spice Keto Cookies

Day 56

Breakfast: Greek Yogurt and Walnut Parfait

Lunch: Spinach and Artichoke Stuffed Chicken

Dinner: Creamy Spinach and Mushroom Stuffed Pork Tenderloin

Snack: Chocolate Mint Avocado Pudding

Day 57

Breakfast: Creamy Avocado and Smoked Salmon Toast

Lunch: Salmon and Avocado Salad

Dinner: Keto Beef Stroganoff

Snack: Cacao Nib and Almond Butter Cups

Day 58

Breakfast: Keto Veggie and Cheese Frittata Muffins

Lunch: Creamy Spinach and Artichoke Stuffed Chicken Breasts

Dinner: Lemon Butter Baked Cod with Herbed Tomatoes

Snack: Keto Peanut Butter Fudge

Day 59

Breakfast: Cinnamon Coconut Porridge

Lunch: Shrimp and Cauliflower Rice Stir-Fry

Dinner: Stuffed Zucchini Boats with Ground Turkey

Snack: Coconut Lime Energy Bites

Day 60 (Final Day)

Breakfast: Blueberry Chia Pudding

Lunch: Thai Coconut Chicken Soup

Dinner: Keto Pesto and Mozzarella Stuffed Chicken

Snack: Keto Cheesecake Bites

<u>Congratulations On Completing The 60-Day Keto Meal Plan!</u>

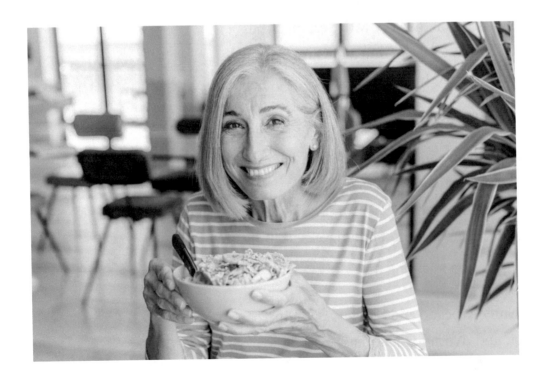

By now, you should have adapted to this eating pattern and experienced its potential benefits. Remember to continue making mindful food choices and listening to your body's needs.

Below, you'll find a summary of useful tips that we've covered throughout the book for all of you, women over 70:

- ✓ **Stay Hydrated:** Aging can reduce the sensation of thirst, so make a conscious effort to drink enough water daily.

- ✓ **Maintain Muscle Mass:** Regular exercise, especially strength training, can help preserve muscle mass and strength.

- ✓ **Monitor Bone Health:** Regular check-ups for bone density and supplements when necessary are crucial for healthy bones.

- ✓ **Mindful Eating:** Pay attention to portion sizes and avoid mindless snacking.

- ✓ **Consult a Healthcare Professional:** Before making significant dietary changes, it's advisable to consult with a healthcare provider, especially if you have underlying health conditions.

- ✓ **Grocery Shopping:** Opt for fresh, whole foods, and prioritize organic and locally sourced options whenever possible.

- ✓ **Listen to Your Body:** Your body's nutritional needs can change with age, so stay attuned to your body's signals and make adjustments as needed.

- ✓ **Social Connection:** Maintaining social relationships and staying engaged with family and friends is vital for emotional well-being.

- ✓ **Regular Health Screenings:** Schedule regular check-ups to detect and address health issues early, including eye and dental exams.

- ✓ **Mental Wellness:** Prioritize mental health through activities like meditation, mindfulness, or hobbies you enjoy.

- ✓ **Sleep Quality:** Ensure you get sufficient and restful sleep to support overall health and energy levels.

- ✓ **Eye Health:** Regular eye exams are vital, as eye health can deteriorate with age. Consider foods rich in lutein and zeaxanthin, like leafy greens, to support eye health.

Keto Diet for Women Over 70 Guided Nutrition Tracker

Name:

Start Date of Tracking:

Keto Diet Goal:

Ketosis Level:

Monitor and record your ketosis level daily using keto test strips.

Day 1

Ketosis Level:

Notes:

Day 2

Ketosis Level:

Notes:

...

Nutrition Intake

Log the meals and snacks you consume. Pay attention to portion sizes and the quality of foods you choose.

Day 1

Meal 1:

Meal 2:

Snack:

Meal 3:

Notes:

Day 2

Meal 1:

Meal 2:

Snack:

Meal 3:

Notes:

...

Non-Scale Victories

Every day, write down the non-scale victories you experienced thanks to the ketogenic diet. These could include improved digestion, reduced cravings, enhanced focus, or healthier skin.

Day 1

Non-Scale Victory:

Notes:

...

Day 2

Non-Scale Victory:

Notes:

Energy and Well-being

Monitor your energy levels and overall well-being throughout the day. Take note of any variations or changes you noticed.

Day 1

Energy Levels:

General Well-being:

Notes:

Day 2

Energy Levels:

General Well-being:

Notes:

...

Physical Changes

Occasionally, take time to evaluate any physical changes related to the ketogenic diet. These may include changes in weight, measurements, or body composition.

Day 1

Weight:

Measurements:

Body Composition:

Notes:

Day 2

Weight:

Measurements:

Body Composition:

Notes:

...

Guided Roadmap for the Keto Diet

These guides will help you track your ketogenic diet progress in a structured and mindful way. Be patient with yourself, as individual responses may vary. Tailor the keto diet to your individual needs and experiment till you find the best routine for your journey.

Step 1: Choose Your Tracker

Select the tracking method that suits you best: pen and paper, mobile app, or smartwatch/fitness tracker.

Step 2: Clear Goals

Clearly define your keto diet goals, like achieving and maintaining ketosis, weight management, enhanced energy, or improved mental clarity.

Step 3: Ketosis Level Monitoring

Record and monitor your ketosis level daily using keto test strips to ensure you're in a state of ketosis.

Step 4: Mindful Eating

Monitor your food intake, ensuring you make nutritious and balanced choices following the Keto Diet for Women Over 70.

Step 5: Non-Scale Victories

Recognize victories unrelated to the scale, like improved sleep, reduced inflammation, or an improved mood.

Step 6: Energy and Well-being

Be mindful of your energy levels throughout the day and how the ketogenic diet impacts your overall well-being.

Step 7: Physical Changes

Occasionally evaluate any physical changes, but remember that progress may be gradual and vary from person to person.

Step 8: Reflection and Adaptation

Weekly, reflect on your progress and adapt your ketogenic diet routine based on results and personal needs.

Step 9: Celebrate Success

Celebrate your successes and small victories along the ketogenic diet journey to keep motivation high.

Conclusion

As we conclude this journey through the world of the ketogenic diet for women over 70, it's vital to reflect on the key concepts and the invaluable insights we've explored together. The path to healthy aging is paved with choices, and embracing the ketogenic lifestyle can be a transformational one.

Throughout this book, we've delved into the changes that naturally occur in our bodies as we age and how the ketogenic diet plays a pivotal role in helping us age gracefully. We've discovered the nuances of achieving and maintaining ketosis safely, and the various forms of the ketogenic diet that can be tailored to suit the unique needs of older women. Balancing diet with lifestyle, overcoming challenges, and navigating potential risks and side effects have been at the core of our discussions.

The benefits of the ketogenic diet for women over 70 are abundant. From supporting bone health to promoting heart health, this lifestyle choice can truly enhance the quality of life. It's a journey that empowers us to maintain a healthy weight, sustain muscle mass, and enjoy optimal nutrition.

I encourage every woman over 70 to embark on this ketogenic journey with enthusiasm and care. The advantages for your health and well-being are evident, and you are not alone in this path. Many women worldwide have already embraced this lifestyle, forming a supportive community that celebrates the joys of healthy aging through the ketogenic diet.

With mindful eating, regular exercise, and the guidance provided in this book, you are well-equipped to embrace the ketogenic diet and its remarkable potential. The path to a healthier, more vibrant you starts here, and the benefits are waiting for you to seize. Embrace this transformative journey, and may it bring you health, vitality, and the joy of aging gracefully.